Essentials of Airway Management

To our teachers

Essentials of Airway Management

Editor

Sylva Dolenska MD, FRCA
Consultant Anaesthetist
William Harvey Hospital
Ashford, Kent

Authors

Priti Dalal MD, FRCA
Specialist Anaesthetic Registrar
Guy's & St Thomas' Hospital NHS Trust, London

Andrew Taylor BSc, MB BS, FRCA
Specialist Anaesthetic Registrar
South East Thames Rotation

www.greenwich-medical.co.uk

© 2004
Greenwich Medical Media Limited
137 Euston Road
London
NW1 2AA

870 Market St, Ste 720
San Francisco, CA 94102

ISBN 184 110 1532

First Published 2004

A catalogue record for this book is available from the British Library

Typeset by Mizpah Publishing Services, Chennai, India

Printed in Malta by the Gutenberg Press

Contents

Preface

Airway management is a practical skill. It was traditionally taught in the form of an apprenticeship – 'learning on the job'. Acquiring the practical skill in the operating theatre is still an essential part of the training. However, to my knowledge there is no textbook of basic airway management for the novice trainee. Maintaining the airway is a vital part of the anaesthetist's job: the patient's life depends on it. The novice trainee is expected to be competent at basic airway management, including anaesthesia and its complications, after only three months of training. This book provides concise and basic information; it only briefly mentions advanced or specialist techniques. It is hoped that it will prove useful for the anaesthetic senior house officers (SHOs) and operating department assistants.

Sylva Dolenska

January 2004

Foreword

I wish this volume had been available when I was starting anaesthesia. Sylva Dolenska and her colleagues set themselves a formidable task. We all know that it is easier to write at length than concisely. To be brief, inclusive and clear is difficult, but in my view they have succeeded. There will always be different opinions on the 'best' way of doing virtually everything, so most experienced anaesthetists will doubtless find points they disagree with. However, the advice given by Dr Dolenska and her colleagues is down to earth, as befits their background in busy clinical environments, and can be followed with confidence by inexperienced practitioners.

Mortality from airway problems during anaesthesia is rare these days, but the level of anxiety exhibited by anaesthetists has not decreased, indeed most of us are more anxious than we used to be, because of a perceived, and probably actual, increase in medico-legal vulnerability. Nevertheless, such serenity as can be reasonably expected during an anaesthetic career comes with the acquisition of knowledge. This book will be a portable, sensible source of knowledge and advice for trainee anaesthetists.

Ian Calder
Consultant Anaesthetist to
The National Hospital for Neurology and
Neurosurgery and The Royal Free Hospital

Acknowledgement

I would like to thank my proof readers, Dr. Nichola White and Dr. Alison Macdonald, for their helpful comments and suggestions.

Sylva Dolenska

ACKNOWLEDGEMENT

Chapter 1

Airway Assessment

Sylva Dolenska

An inadequate airway leads rapidly to hypoxaemia and uncorrected hypoxaemia will result in brain damage and ultimately death. The object of the ideal airway assessment test is to anticipate possible problems with the planned technique of airway management. The 'gold standard' for a secure airway is tracheal intubation. Therefore, even if the planned technique does not involve tracheal intubation, every airway assessment should include tests that aim to predict difficulty with tracheal intubation.

There are many anatomical and physiological factors that influence the ease of laryngoscopy and intubation. No single test can predict airway or intubation difficulty reliably. The ability to detect an abnormality (to detect true positives) is described as the *sensitivity* of a test. The ability to differentiate between abnormality and normal (to reject false positives) is the *specifity* of the test. The ability to identify the false negatives is described as its *positive predictive value*. No single test, or a combination of tests, can detect difficulty with airway management with 100% certainty. When combining tests, specificity and positive predictive value improve, while sensitivity decreases. However, a combination of unfavourable features will alert the anaesthetist to a higher probability of difficulty, so that preparations can be made.

Bedside assessment
For a systematic bedside approach to assess the airway, the acronym '**MOUTHS**' has been proposed by Davies and Eagle, which may be a useful mnemotechnic for the trainee anaesthetist. The letters stand for: **M**andible, **O**pening, **U**vula, **T**eeth, **H**ead and neck, **S**ilhouette.

Mandible
Assess mandibular length (measure mental-thyroid distance) and grade of mandibular protrusion (jaw thrust).

Jaw protrusion (Figure 1.1) is a useful test, as it indicates the ability to displace the tongue anteriorly. Patients may have difficulty in understanding what is required; try a demonstration or ask them to bite the upper lip. Full protrusion (lower incisors anterior to upper incisors) is classed as class A, part protrusion (upper and lower incisors in line) as class B, no protrusion (lower incisors behind upper) as class C.

Mento-thyroid distance depends on which point on the chin is taken as the starting point. Various criteria have been proposed; a distance of less than 6 cm (approximately the width of the examiner's fingers 2–5) is found in individuals with a small receding mandible, Pierre-Robin syndrome etc.

Opening
The *gape* should be at least 3 cm, in order to accommodate the laryngoscope blade. The width of three examiner's fingers is usually more

AIRWAY ASSESSMENT

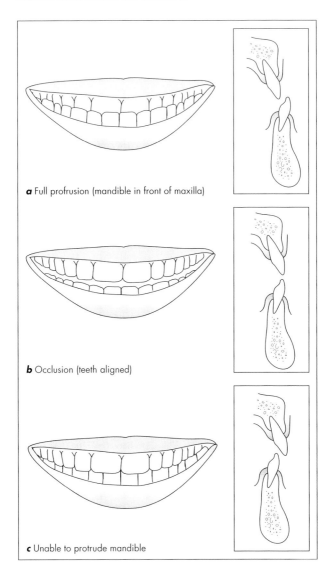

a Full profrusion (mandible in front of maxilla)

b Occlusion (teeth aligned)

c Unable to protrude mandible

Figure 1.1 Jaw protrusion.

than this distance, while the width of two fingers usually signifies a problem with mouth opening. This problem may be due to muscle spasm or temporo-mandibular joint disease. Muscle spasm can usually (but not always) be overcome by relaxation under general anaesthesia; temporo-mandibular arthritis may cause severe functional or anatomical limit to mouth opening that does not improve with muscle relaxation.

Uvula (including the palate and the pharyngeal structures)
The visibility of the uvula after maximum mouth opening with tongue protrusion is a part of a system of classification originally proposed by Mallampati and modified by Samsoon and Young. Although anaesthetists now commonly use the term 'Mallampati grade I to IV' (Figure 1.2a), this is a misnomer as in fact the original *Mallampati scoring* was based on three classes: what we use now is the modification by Samsoon and Young depicted in Figure 1.2, but the name Mallampati continues to be used. Notice that hardly any (class III) or no (class IV) posterior pharyngeal wall can be seen in the two higher classes. Even with best standardisation (patient sitting, head in neutral position, maximum mouth opening and tongue protrusion – Figure 1.2b) there is inter-observer variability and a relatively high incidence of false negatives. Assess also the shape of the palate – a high arched palate is associated with several congenital anomalies of the airway. Note that higher grades of Mallampati do not necessarily correlate with higher grades at laryngoscopy (see Chapter 3: Routine Intubation).

Teeth
Assess presence of loose or decayed teeth, crowns, gaps and dental appliances. A completely edentulous patient has a wider gape and therefore is relatively easy to intubate. A complete set of healthy teeth rarely presents a problem but a gap in the right upper quadrant may, as the laryngoscope blade has a tendency to slip in this gap. Damaged teeth, particularly in front, may be in danger of dislocation or trauma with the laryngoscope blade. Caps or crowns are expensive to replace and should be protected from damage. Ask the patient to remove their partial denture to see gaps; for intubation, a well fitting partial denture may be left in situ to prevent problems with gaps but take care with the laryngoscope.

Head
Assess all ranges of *movement* of the head (atlanto-occipital joint) and cervical spine. Full atlanto-occipital and cervical spine mobility will achieve at least a 90° difference between full flexion (chin on chest) and extension (ask the patient to look at the ceiling while sitting upright). This is a useful test as the absence of movement particularly in the atlanto-occipital joint may make it physically impossible to

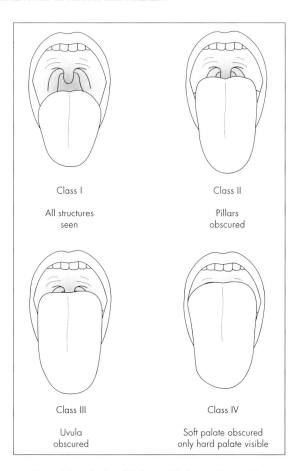

Class I

All structures
seen

Class II

Pillars
obscured

Class III

Uvula
obscured

Class IV

Soft palate obscured
only hard palate visible

Figure 1.2 a Grades of Mallampati (Redrawn with permission
from Ellis H, Feldman S. *Anatomy for Anaesthetists*, 7th edn.
Blackwell Publishing Ltd, 1996).

obtain a line of vision at attempted direct laryngoscopy. (The line
joining the upper incisors and the base of the tongue in this case does
not align with the midline axis of the larynx and the trachea.) The
movement is best observed from profile; sufficient head extension
occurs if the chin reaches a point higher with respect to the occiput
than in neutral position (Delilkan) – Figure 1.3.

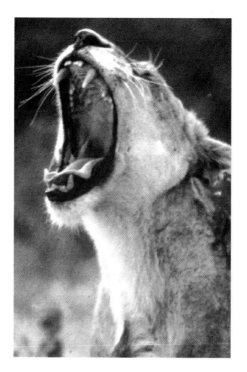

Figure 1.2 b Lion's mouth – ideal mouth opening
(Courtesy of Dr. Ian Calder)

AIRWAY ASSESSMENT

Silhouette
Assess the profile of the head, neck and chest. Notice receding chin – Figure 1.4 ('chinless wonder'), swellings or tumours in the neck, short or absent neck, acromegalic facies, kyphosis, in particular in ankylosing spondylitis and large breasts. These features may present a problem at intubation. Facemask ventilation is difficult in patients with beards and often also in edentulous elderly patients, due to the difficulty in maintaining a seal with a facemask.

To this the author would also add another 'S': *Stridor* – a sign that signifies severe narrowing of the upper airway and another 'H' for *History* – enquire about problems with breathing under previous anaesthetics and examine old notes for anaesthetic records, ITU admissions, X-rays etc. Patients with upper airway tumours or neck masses need to be re-assessed each time they present for surgery: a compromised upper airway is a threat to life. Difficult airway is dealt with in Chapter 11: The Difficult Airway.

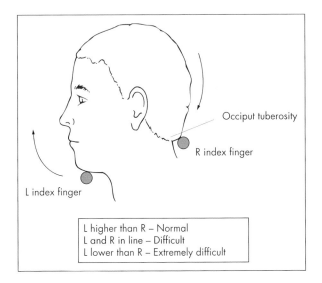

Occiput tuberosity

R index finger

L index finger

L higher than R – Normal
L and R in line – Difficult
L lower than R – Extremely difficult

Figure 1.3 Delilkan sign.

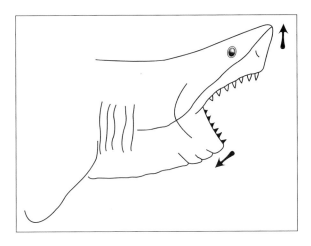

Figure 1.4 Receding chin (No problem in a shark as it does not have or need an airway). Picture supplied courtesy of Dr. Ian Calder

The combination of Mallampati, jaw protrusion and craniocervical extension has a specificity of 99% and positive predictive value of 93%. This is at the expense of a lower sensitivity. In other words, a patient who is identified as possibly difficult will in all likelihood be difficult; however, some cases classified as 'easy' will be only identified at laryngoscopy as 'difficult'.

Radiological assessment

Many tests and measurements have been described but few offer additional information to the bedside tests outlined above. In rheumatoid arthritis with cervical spine involvement X-rays and magnetic resonance imaging (MRI) of cervical spine should be obtained to establish a diagnosis of cervical spine instability.

In patients with hoarseness or stridor, when possible, a computed tomogram (CT) of the laryngeal inlet and trachea will allow assessment of the degree of the upper airway narrowing. This will help the selection of an appropriate size of tracheal tube.

After assessing the airway, form a plan for airway management. Specific situations will be discussed in the next chapters.

Summary

A thorough bedside assessment of the airway will alert the anaesthetist to most cases of difficulties with laryngoscopy and intubation. However, some cases will only be discovered at intubation.

Bibliography

Cormack RS, Lehane J. Difficult tracheal intubation in obstetrics. *Anaesthesia* 1984; 39: 1105–1111.

Wilson ME. Predicting difficult intubation. *BJA* 1993; 71: 333–334.

Yentis S. Predicting difficult intubation – Worthwhile exercise or pointless ritual. *Anaesthesia* 2002; 57: 105–109.

Davies JM, Eagle CJ. MOUTHS. *Can J Anaesth.* 1991; 38: 687.

AIRWAY ASSESSMENT

Chapter 2

Anatomy

Priti Dalal

This chapter describes the key elements of the anatomy of the airway that are of relevance to the trainee anaesthetist.

Mouth

The mouth extends from the lips to the palatoglossal arches. It is divided anatomically into two parts – the vestibule and the mouth cavity. The narrow space between the lips, cheek, teeth and gums is the vestibule of the mouth. The mouth cavity is the space inner to the teeth and the gums. Its floor is formed by the tongue and the roof by the hard palate.

Applied anatomy
1. Oropharyngeal airway and oral intubation are commonly used as a means to maintain the patency of the airway.
2. Several tests are used to predict a difficult airway – e.g. mouth opening, jaw subluxation and Mallampati score. These are described in Chapter 1: Airway Assessment.
3. Trauma to the lips, teeth (especially to caps and crowns) and tongue can occur when laryngoscopy is difficult, so the practitioner should be gentle while performing this procedure.

Nose

Anatomically, the nose can be divided into two parts: the external nose and the nasal cavity. The nasal cavity is divided into two halves – the right and the left – by a nasal septum in the midline (Figure 2.1).

The external nose projects from the face and consists of the nasal bones and cartilages. These are covered by fibroadipose tissue and the skin. Its blood supply is from the dorsal nasal (ophthalmic), external nasal (from anterior ethmoidal), lateral nasal (facial) and septal (superior labial) arteries.

The nasal cavity extends from the nostrils to the posterior end of the nasal septum. It is pear-shaped on cross-section. It opens into the nasopharynx through the posterior nasal apertures. It consists of three areas:

- *Respiratory area* – occupies most of the cavity and is lined by pseudostratified ciliated columnar epithelium.
- *Vestibular area* – this is just inside the nostril and is lined by skin.
- *Olfactory area* – this occupies the uppermost part of the nasal septum and lateral wall over the superior conchae. It contains receptors for the special sense of smell.

The floor of the nose is formed by the hard palate. The nasal septum consists of the vomer, the perpendicular plate of the ethmoid and the septal cartilage. The lateral wall of the nose is formed (from above

ANATOMY

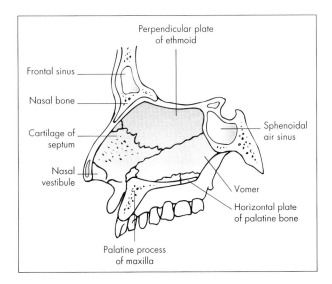

Figure 2.1 Nasal septum (Redrawn with permission from Ellis H, Feldman S. *Anatomy for Anaesthetists*, 7th edn. Blackwell Publishing Ltd, 1996).

downwards) by the medial wall of the orbit and the medial wall of the maxillary sinus. There are three conchae (turbinates) that project into the nasal cavity.

Blood supply
The sphenopalatine artery is the main artery supplying the mucosa over the conchae, the meati and much of the septum. On the lower anterior part of the septum (Little's area), it anastomoses with the septal branch of the superior labial and the ascending branch of the greater palatine. This forms the Kiesselbach's plexus, which is a common site for epistaxis.

Nerve supply
- Olfactory area – olfactory nerves (I)
- Vestibular area – infra-orbital nerve (V_1)
- Respiratory area – anterior dental branch, nasopalatine and anterior palatine nerves (V_2)

With the exception of the olfactory nerves, all are branches of the trigeminal nerve, its first and second division (ophthalmic and superior maxillary nerve).

Applied anatomy

Nasal intubation is frequently carried out for dental and maxillo-facial surgery. The nose has a rich blood supply; hence trauma during nasal intubation can cause bleeding. One needs to look for enlarged inferior turbinates, deviated septum or septal spur before inserting the naso-tracheal tube through that particular nostril.

Palate

This has two parts – the hard and the soft palate. The hard palate is made up of the palatal process of the maxilla and the horizontal plate of the palatine bone. The soft palate is a mass of soft tissue that hangs from the posterior edge of the hard palate as a mobile fold. It fuses with the lateral wall of the pharynx at the sides. During swallowing, its lower border makes contact with the posterior pharyngeal wall, thereby closing off the nasopharynx. It is made up of a tough fibrous sheath called the palatine aponeurosis which is attached to the poster-ior edge of the hard palate and is continuous on each side with the tendon of the tensor palati.

The soft palate is made up of five muscles:
1. Tensor veli palate – tightens and flattens the soft palate
2. Levator palati – elevates the soft palate
3. Palatoglossus – approximates the palatoglossal folds
4. Palatopharyngeus – approximates the palatopharyngeal folds
5. Musculus uvulae

Sensory nerve supply is from the maxillary division of the trigeminal nerve. Motor supply for the tensor palati is from mandibular division of the trigeminal nerve. The rest of the palatine muscles are innervated from the pharyngeal plexus which transmits cranial fibres of the accessory nerve via the vagus. The soft palate acts as a flap valve that can shut off the oropharynx from the mouth during chewing or from the nasopharynx during swallowing and coughing.

Pharynx

The pharynx is essentially a common upper pathway for the respiratory and alimentary tracts. It is a fibromuscular tube extending downwards from the base of the skull to the level of the C6 vertebra – it then continues as the oesophagus. It is deficient anteriorly where it com-municates with the nose, mouth and larynx, thereby forming the nasopharynx, oropharynx and the laryngopharynx respectively. The wall of the pharynx consists of four layers which, from the innermost out, are the mucosa, the submucous fibrous layer, muscle and the buccopharyngeal fascia.

The muscular layer consists of three sheets of muscles – the superior, middle and inferior constrictors. The muscles overlap posteriorly and

ANATOMY

are telescoped into each other like three stacked cups. These muscles are supplemented by the stylopharyngeus, palatopharyngeus and the salpingopharyngeus.

Nasopharynx
The nasopharynx lies behind the nasal cavity, above the soft palate. It communicates with the oropharynx through the pharyngeal isthmus. The pharyngeal opening of the Eustachian tube lies behind and just below the inferior nasal concha. On the roof and the posterior wall of the nasopharynx lie the adenoids. At the base of the skull, the wall of the nasopharynx consists of a rigid membrane – the pharyngo-basilar fascia.

Oropharynx
The mouth communicates with the pharynx through the oropharyn-geal isthmus. This is bounded by the palatoglossal arches, the soft palate and the dorsum of the tongue. The oropharynx extends from the soft palate to the tip of the epiglottis. The palatine tonsil is a large collection of lymphoid tissue which projects into the oropharynx from the tonsillar fossa, the triangular area between the palatopharyngeal fold behind and the palatoglossal fold in front. The mucosa over the tonsil is supplied by the tonsillar branch of the glossopharyngeal nerve and the lesser palatine nerves.

The valleculae are the shallow pits that lie between the epiglottis and the posterior part of the tongue. They are separated by the median glosso-epiglottic fold in the midline and the lateral glosso-epiglottic folds inferolaterally.

Laryngopharynx
This extends from the upper border of the epiglottis to the level of the cricoid cartilage (C6) vertebra where it becomes continuous with the oesophagus.

The main features are the laryngeal inlet and the piriform recesses on either side. The lateral glosso-epiglottic folds on either side separate the oral from the laryngeal part of the pharynx. Below this are the piriform fossae. The posterior wall is formed by the three overlapping constrictor muscles up to the level of the vocal cords. Below this are the Killian's dehiscence and the cricopharyngeal sphincter.

Nerve supply of the pharynx
Motor
All the muscles of the pharynx are supplied by the pharyngeal plexus except the stylopharyngeus, which is supplied by the glossopharyngeal nerve. The pharyngeal plexus is formed by the union of the pharyngeal branches from the vagus, glossopharyngeal and the cervical sympathetic nerves.

ANATOMY

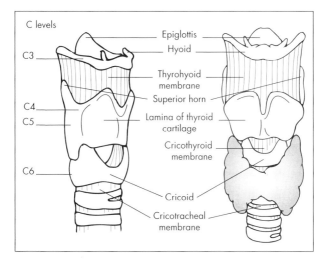

Figure 2.2 External view of the larynx (Redrawn with permission from Ellis H, Feldman S. *Anatomy for Anaesthetists*, 7th edn. Blackwell Publishing Ltd, 1996).

ANATOMY

Sensory
• Nasopharynx – maxillary nerve (from the trigeminal).
• Oropharynx – glossopharyngeal nerve, valleculae – internal laryngeal nerve (vagus).
• Laryngopharynx – internal and recurrent laryngeal nerve.

Larynx
The larynx or the sound-box is in the part of the respiratory tract between the pharynx and the trachea. It lies below the hyoid bone in the midline of the neck extending from the C3 to the C6 vertebra (Figure 2.2).

The larynx consists of
1. Cartilages (paired and unpaired)
   • *Paired* – arytenoids, corniculate and cuneiform
   • *Unpaired* – thyroid, cricoid and epiglottic
2. Joints – cricothyroid, cricoarytenoid and arytenocorniculate
3. Ligaments and membranes – these can be classified as extrinsic (thyrohyoid membrane, cricotracheal and hyoepiglottic ligaments) and intrinsic (quadrangular membrane, cricothyroid ligament)
4. Muscles

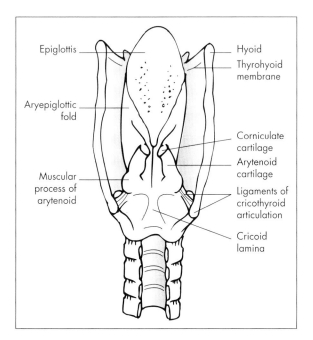

Figure 2.3 Cartilages and membranes of the larynx in section (Redrawn with permission from Ellis H, Feldman S. *Anatomy for Anaesthetists*, 7th edn. Blackwell Publishing Ltd, 1996).

1. Cartilages (Figure 2.3)
Thyroid cartilage: This is shield-like, made of two conjoined laminae the union of which anteriorly forms the pharyngeal prominence or the Adam's apple. It has a free posterior border which projects upwards and downwards as the superior and the inferior cornu. The inferior horns articulate with the cricoid cartilage to form the cricothyroid joint.

Cricoid cartilage: This is a signet ring-shaped structure to which the thyroid and the arytenoid cartilages are articulated. It is the only complete cartilaginous ring in the whole of the air passage. It consists of a narrow arch anteriorly and a quadrangular flat part posteriorly.

Epiglottic cartilage: This is a slightly curled, leaf-shaped structure which overhangs the vestibule of the larynx. Its upper border is attached in the midline to the thyroid cartilage.

ANATOMY

Arytenoid cartilages: These are pyramid-shaped cartilages, one on either side. Each has a vocal process at the base which is attached to the vocal folds and a lateral projection called the muscular process to which the cricoarytenoid muscle is attached. The superior process articulates with the corniculate cartilages on either side. The aryepiglottic fold is attached to the corniculate cartilages. The inferior surface articulates with the upper border of the cricoid cartilage forming the crico-arytenoid joint.

The corniculate and the cuneiform cartilages make the small whitish elevations on top and in front of the arytenoids.

2. Joints

Cricothyroid joint: This is a synovial joint formed between the inferior horn of the thyroid cartilage and the facet on the cricoid. The movement between the two joints is such that one cartilage can rock over the other.

Cricoarytenoid joint: This is formed between the cricoid cartilage and the inferior surface of the arytenoids cartilage. The rotary and gliding movements along these joints allows the rima glottidis (gap between the vocal cords), to be opened in a 'v' or diamond shape.

3. Ligaments and membranes (Figure 2.3)

Extrinsic membranes and ligaments are those connecting the larynx to structures above (i.e. to the hyoid) and below (i.e. to the trachea). There are three of these:

- The thyrohyoid membrane
- The cricotracheal ligament
- The hyoepiglottic ligament

The *thyrohyoid membrane* extends from the upper border of the thyroid cartilage to the upper border of the hyoid bone. It has a thickening in the midline called the median thyrohyoid ligament. The posterior free borders form the lateral thyrohyoid ligament. This membrane forms the lateral wall of the piriform fossa. It suspends the larynx on the hyoid bone.

The *cricotracheal ligament* is made of fibrous tissue similar to the membrane that connects the rings of the trachea.

The *hyoepiglottic ligament* is an elastic band from the anterior surface of the epiglottis to the hyoid.

Some texts also include the *cricothyroid ligament*, although this is strictly speaking an internal ligament, interconnecting the laryngeal cartilages.

ANATOMY

Intrinsic membranes and ligaments (those interconnecting the cartilages of the larynx) are numerous; below are those of significance for the anaesthetist.

The *cricothyroid membrane* extends from the upper border of the cricoid cartilage to the lower border of the thyroid cartilage. It is subcutaneous in the midline and thus accessible to needling for surgical access to the airway.

The epiglottis is connected to the sides of the arytenoid cartilages via the *quadrangular membrane*, which forms the frame of the aryepiglottic folds. It is attached to the tongue by the median *glosso-epiglottic folds* and to the pharynx by the lateral glosso-epiglottic folds.

4. Muscles
These can be divided into intrinsic and extrinsic.

There are nine *intrinsic muscles* of the larynx and they are divided into:
1. Those that alter the *size and the shape of the laryngeal inlet* – aryepiglottic, oblique arytenoids, thyroepiglottic (depressor epiglottidis) muscle
2. Those that *move the vocal cords* – these can be divided into adductors and abductors:
   - *Adductors* – lateral cricoarytenoid, transverse arytenoids
   - *Abductors* – posterior cricoarytenoid
3. Those that regulate the *tension of the vocal cords*:
   - *Cricothyroid* – tenses and lengthens the vocal cords
   - *Thyroarytenoid* – relaxes and shortens the vocal cords
   - *Vocalis* – thin band in the vocal cord

The principal *extrinsic muscles* are the sternothyroid, which depresses the larynx and the thyrohyoid, which elevates it. Other extrinsic muscles are attached to the hyoid.

The cavity of the larynx (Figure 2.4)
The inlet of the larynx faces backwards and upwards. It is anteriorly bounded by the upper edge of the epiglottis, posteriorly by the mucous membrane stretched between the arytenoids and laterally by the aryepiglottic fold. The space below the level of the inlet up to the vestibular folds is called the *vestibule*. The superior or *false vocal cords* (also known as vestibular folds) are not concerned with voice production. They are two thick folds of mucous membrane, enclosing a narrow band of fibrous tissue, the superior thyroarytenoid ligament. The *ventricle* or the *sinus* of the larynx is an oblong fossa between the true and false vocal cords. The true cords are the thickened edge of the cricovocal membrane.

ANATOMY

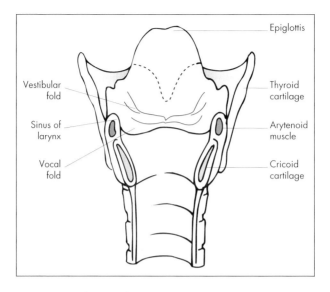

Figure 2.4 The cavity of the larynx in transverse section (Redrawn with permission from Ellis H, Feldman S. *Anatomy for Anaesthetists*, 7th edn. Blackwell Publishing Ltd, 1996).

The *rima glottidis* is an anteroposterior slit. The anterior 60% is bounded on each side by the vocal cords. The posterior 40% on each side is formed by the vocal process of the arytenoid cartilages.

Nerve supply of the larynx (Figure 2.5)
The nerve supply of the larynx is by branches of the superior laryngeal nerve (external and internal) and the recurrent (inferior) laryngeal nerve. All these are branches of the *vagus nerve* (X).

Sensory supply
Sensory supply above the level of the vocal cords is by the internal laryngeal nerve. It pierces the thyrohyoid membrane above the superior laryngeal artery. It can be blocked at this point below the greater cornu of the hyoid.

Below the level of the vocal cords the laryngeal sensory supply is by the recurrent laryngeal nerve.

Motor supply
The recurrent laryngeal nerve supplies all the intrinsic muscles of the larynx except the cricothyroid, which is supplied by the external laryngeal nerve.

ANATOMY

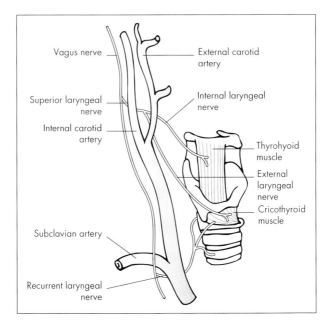

Figure 2.5 The nerve supply of the larynx (From Erdmann A. *Concise Anatomy for Anaesthesia*. Greenwich Medical Media Ltd, 2001).

ANATOMY

Trachea

The trachea is a continuation of the larynx. It starts in the neck below the cricoid cartilage, at the level of the C6 vertebra. The cricotracheal ligament attaches it to the lower margin of the cricoid cartilage. The tracheal wall is made up of C-shaped incomplete cartilages called tracheal rings. Posteriorly there lies a gap in this ring which is filled by the trachealis muscle. The fibrous tissue has a high content of elastic fibres to facilitate the elastic recoil, which is necessary during respiration. The mucosa consists of pseudostratified columnar ciliated epithelium. The total length of the trachea is 10–11 cm but during deep inspiration this may increase to 14–15 cm. It enters the thoracic inlet in the midline. It passes downwards, dividing into two main bronchi; the cartilage dividing the bronchi is the carina.

Anatomically, the trachea can be divided into two parts – the *cervical* and the *thoracic*.

The cervical part lies anterior to the oesophagus in the neck. The recurrent laryngeal nerve lies in the tracheo-oesophageal groove.

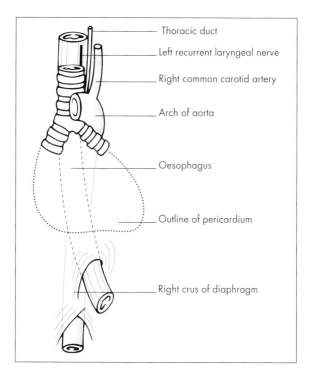

- Thoracic duct
- Left recurrent laryngeal nerve
- Right common carotid artery
- Arch of aorta
- Oesophagus
- Outline of pericardium
- Right crus of diaphragm

ANATOMY

Figure 2.6 Trachea and its relations in the mediastinum (Redrawn with permission from Ellis H, Feldman S. *Anatomy for Anaesthetists*, 7th edn. Blackwell Publishing Ltd, 1996).

Laterally, the trachea is related to the carotid sheath. At the level of the second, third and fourth cervical ring, the thyroid isthmus is related anteriorly, the lobes of the thyroid gland extending as far down as the sixth tracheal ring.

The thoracic part of the trachea runs through the superior mediastinum anterior to the oesophagus. In the thorax, the trachea is related to several important structures (Figure 2.6).

Blood supply is by inferior thyroid and bronchial arteries, venous drainage by the inferior thyroid plexus, lymphatic drainage via the deep cervical and the paratracheal lymph nodes.

Nerve supply: The mucosa is supplied by the vagus and the recurrent laryngeal nerve.

Applied anatomy

The cricothyroid membrane is a commonly used site to carry out a 'needle cricothyroidotomy' or a laryngotomy. This is a life saving measure in a 'cannot intubate cannot ventilate situation'. This technique is a part of advanced airway management and is described elsewhere in the book.

Anaesthesia for awake fibreoptic intubation of the airway

Note: This is a technique for advanced airway management, included here only for interest.

The nose and the nasopharynx

Lignocaine 10% spray, which delivers 10 mg per dose, may be sprayed in each nostril. A lignocaine nebuliser may also be used. A 2% lignocaine gel has the advantage of being a topical anaesthetic as well as a lubricant.

As the nose is very vascular, there is an increased chance of bleeding thereby making visualisation through the endoscope difficult. A vasoconstrictor such as phenylephrine 0.25–1% nasal drops or xylometazoline nasal drops may be used to reduce the risk of bleeding. Cocaine 5–10%, up to 1.5 mg/kg may also be used as it has both local anaesthetic and vasoconstrictor effect. However, it carries the risk of arrhythmias, cardiac ischaemia and central nervous system stimulation associated with its use.

Tongue and the oropharynx

The sensory supply to the posterior one-third of the tongue is by the glossopharyngeal nerve. The sensory supply to the anterior two-third of the tongue is by the lingual branch of the mandibular division of the trigeminal nerve. 10% lignocaine spray is used. Alternatively, viscous lignocaine gargles may be used.

Laryngopharynx and larynx: 'spray-as-you' go technique

A syringe containing lignocaine 4% topical (40 mg/ml) is attached to the injection port of the fibreoptic laryngoscope. While the patient takes deep breaths, 2 ml is sprayed on the epiglottis and about 6 ml on the glottis. Once the glottis is entered, spray another 2 ml of the local anaesthetic solution. The local anaesthetic stimulates the cough reflex which helps the spread of the local anaesthetic solution. This technique is now commonly used.

The nerve blocks are described below.

Glossopharyngeal nerve block

The glossopharyngeal nerve supplies sensation to the posterior one-third of the tongue, the pharynx and the superior surface of the

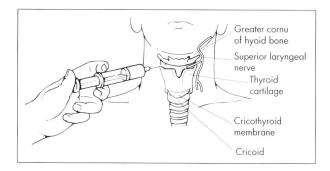

Figure 2.7 Superior laryngeal nerve block (Redrawn with permission from Mulroy MF. *Regional Anaesthesia: An Illustrated Procedural Guide.* © Lippincott, Williams & Wilkins, 1996).

epiglottis. This is blocked on either side by injecting 5 ml of 1–2% lignocaine with a 23 G needle in the area where the base of the tongue opposes the palatoglossal folds. Careful aspiration before injection is important as it is in close proximity to the carotid artery.

Superior laryngeal nerve block (Figure 2.7)
This anaesthetises the inferior surface of the epiglottis, up to the vocal cords. The patient is positioned supine with the head extended. This is achieved by injecting on either side 3–6 ml 1% lignocaine between the greater cornu of the hyoid bone and the thyroid cartilage. As the needle passes through the thyrohyoid membrane, a slight loss of resistance is felt and 3 ml of the local anaesthetic is injected superficial and deep to the membrane. Alternatively, surface anaesthesia may be achieved with lignocaine soaked gauze pads inserted in the piriform fossa with Krause's forceps.

This block is contraindicated in the presence of local pathology, abnormal coagulation or in the case of patients who are at risk of aspiration of gastric contents.

Recurrent laryngeal nerve block
This technique – trans-tracheal injection – provides surface anaesthesia of the trachea below the level of the vocal cords. This area is supplied by the recurrent laryngeal nerve.

The patient is positioned supine and the cricothyroid membrane is located. A 20 G cannula attached to a syringe, gently aspirating while injecting, is inserted in the midline. Aspiration of air confirms placement. The needle is withdrawn and 3–4 ml of lignocaine 4% is

ANATOMY

injected through the cannula. This generates severe coughing by the patient, which aids spread within the trachea and onto the vocal cords.

Summary

A detailed knowledge of the anatomy of the upper airway is essential for basic and advanced airway management.

Bibliography

Harold E, Feldman S. The respiratory pathway; in: *Anatomy for Anaesthetists*, 7th edn. Blackwell Publishing Ltd, Part 1, pp 3–75.

McMinn RMH. Head and neck and spine; in: *Last's Anatomy – Regional and Applied*, 9th edn. Churchill Livingstone, Chapter 6, pp 421–505.

ANATOMY

Chapter 3

Routine Intubation

Sylva Dolenska

Passing a cuffed tracheal tube correctly secures the airway, provided no obstruction is below the tip of the tube, and protects the lungs against aspiration of stomach contents.

Indications for tracheal intubation
Limited access to the airway
This may be because the airway is shared between the anaesthetist and the surgeon (procedures on the upper airway), it is within the operating field (ophthalmic or maxillo-facial surgery), or the airway is otherwise inaccessible (prone position, remote procedures such as MRI).

Abdominal or thoracic relaxation required
To ensure good access and successful closure, full relaxation is needed for abdominal, thoracic and cardiac surgery.

Protection from aspiration
Unconscious patients may be at risk of aspiration. Anaesthetised patients are by definition unconscious but if the stomach is empty and indications above and below do not apply, intubation is not necessary.

Patients with a full stomach, including those with delayed stomach emptying and with gastro-oesophageal reflux (e.g. hiatus hernia or morbid obesity) are at increased risk of aspiration of stomach contents. The stomach may be considered empty 2 h after intake of clear fluids and 6 h after intake of food in adults and children, but not in breast-fed infants. Milk contains protein and fat and is therefore considered as food intake; so are milky drinks. Breast milk is more easily digestible and cleared from the stomach after 4 h. Presence of blood in the upper airway is also an indication for tracheal intubation.

Respiratory arrest with or without cardiac arrest
There is a multitude of causes for respiratory or cardiorespiratory arrest but one best way to secure the airway: by tracheal intubation. A compromised airway may have precipitated or contributed to the event.

Only the first two indications will be considered here as 'routine'.

Physiological effects
Passing the laryngoscope and tracheal tube is a strong stimulus to the autonomic nervous system and to suppress it requires a sufficiently deep plane of anaesthesia.

Respiratory effects
The upper airway is supplied by the cranial nerves IX and X. The epiglottis receives nerve supply from both. Straight blade laryngoscopy

ROUTINE INTUBATION

is thought to cause more potent stimulation (both cranial nerves being involved in the reflex response) than using a curved (Macintosh) laryngoscope, which is only advanced as far as the valleculae.

Respiratory effects include increased respiratory drive, laryngospasm and bronchospasm.

The *cardiovascular response* is usually a sympathoadrenal one with tachycardia, hypertension and sometimes dysrhythmias. In children, a vagal response may pre-dominate with bradycardia and salivation.

Central nervous system effects
These include increased intracranial pressure and intraocular pressure (hypertension and drugs used at induction may contribute to this factor).

Preparation
- Assessment – See Chapter 1: Airway Assessment.
- Equipment – Laryngoscopes, bougies, Magill's forceps, plus a selection of facemasks, airways and tracheal tubes of various sizes.

Only instruments used routinely are mentioned here. The reader is referred to more detailed texts (see reference section) and to study the instruments in their own operating department. The fundamental difference (from the point of view of insertion technique) between the straight blade (Magill) and a curved (Macintosh) laryngoscope is highlighted above. In the United Kingdom, most anaesthetists use the curved Macintosh laryngoscope as their first choice, in preference to the straight blade, which is used as a matter of routine by ENT surgeons. For a routine laryngoscopy and intubation, several instruments should be available in case of equipment failure or anatomical variation (e.g. long blade, McCoy with a flexible tip etc.) The Magill laryngoscope was subsequently modified by Miller and Robertshaw and may be referred to as such.

Tracheal tubes
Tubes currently used for tracheal intubation are single use and are mostly made from PVC. There are differences in appearance and stiffness due to changes in the manufacturing process but the material is the same (PVC). Red rubber re-usable tubes are no longer manufactured but may still be seen occasionally. Other materials used include polyurethane and silicone.

The *size* of the tracheal tube is printed on its cover as well as on the tube itself. Tube sizes from 2.5 mm to 10 mm internal diameter are available. Traditionally, the highest diameter possible was advocated, to facilitate laminar flow and therefore low resistance to breathing: 9 mm for a male, 8 mm for a female, 7 mm for an adolescent (see Chapter 6: The Paediatric Airway, for more detail on the paediatric airway). The advantage of a big diameter has to be balanced against the risk of mucosal damage with an oversized tube.

Cuffed tubes are available from size six (size five for microlaryngoscopy tube). The standard tracheal tube has a low volume, high pressure cuff. This is shaped as a balloon and prevents fairly reliably the passage of liquid below the seal. If used for a long time, it may cause tissue oedema and necrosis. For prolonged intubation, a high volume-low pressure cuff is therefore used. This is cylindrical in shape and therefore in contact with a greater area of mucosa at a lower pressure. The cuff is less elastic, may form folds and it does not, therefore, offer such good protection against aspiration as the high pressure-low volume cuff.

Standard tubes come in a standard length and should preferably be cut to size before use: for oral intubation, 24–25 cm will suffice for an average male and 22–23 cm for an average female (adjust by checking the thyromental distance).

Specialised tubes exist for certain types of surgery, e.g. reinforced tubes for extra protection against kinking (in prone position or other situations where head may be moved during surgery), pre-formed south-facing tubes for ENT procedures in the mouth (RAE – Ring, Adair, Elwyn), pre-formed north-facing tubes for nasal intubation in major maxillo-facial work. These tubes are not cut for use. They usually have a mark on them to indicate the ideal depth of insertion (3 cm above the cuff). RAE tubes have a line on them to indicate the level of the lips.

The patient
Sedative *pre-medication* may help to achieve a smooth induction of anaesthesia without sympathoadrenal response, usually associated with coughing, straining and desaturation. Anti-muscarinic agents were important in the age of inhalational ether anaesthesia. For adults and large (>30 kg) children, anti-muscarinic pre-medication is not necessary now, as today's induction agents have better characteristics (see rapid sequence induction in Chapter 4: Abdominal Surgery, for patients at risk of aspiration).

Conduct of routine intubation
Preparation
- Have a skilled anaesthetic assistant present.
- Check all your equipment (machine, suction, airway devices, laryngoscopes) and drugs.
- Attach a capnograph to the breathing system (preferably a sidestream one to keep the bulk of the breathing system to the minimum).

ROUTINE INTUBATION

- Check that rapid head-down tilt can be achieved on the trolley or bed.
- Attach standard monitoring – ECG, pulse oximetry, non-invasive blood pressure.

Induction of anaesthesia
Anaesthetists undertake routine intubation on anaesthetised patients, with or without the aid of neuromuscular relaxation.

The patient is placed supine with one pillow under the head and intravenous access is established. The bed or trolley is raised to a suitable level (according to the anaesthetist's height). Pre-oxygenation is advisable and important in the obese, children or ischaemic heart disease. In these situations, oxygen reserve is diminished, the demands are greater, or both. Emergencies are dealt with elsewhere.

Full *suppression of laryngeal reflexes* is required. This is achieved by intravenous induction and using a neuromuscular blocker, or by deep inhalational anaesthesia. Most patients prefer intravenous induction, while inhalational anaesthesia may be used in paediatrics, the needle-phobic patient, difficult airway, or some emergencies, dealt with elsewhere in this book. After intravenous induction, maintenance must start (oxygen/nitrous oxide/volatile agent or total intravenous anaesthesia).

If using a long-acting neuromuscular blocker, the trainee anaesthetist should make a couple of '*test inflations*' before giving the paralysing agent; if facemask ventilation is proving difficult at this stage, the strategy may be altered (see Chapter 11: The difficult airway). The trainee in such a situation should use suxamethonium as it has the shortest offset time.

Laryngoscopy
When neuromuscular block has set in, perform a laryngoscopy (Figure 3.1). The anaesthetist stands at the head of the bed and holds the laryngoscope in the left hand. The right hand may adjust the position of the head to the 'sniffing the morning air' position, i.e. neck flexed and head (atlanto-occipital joint) extended. The laryngoscope is placed in the right corner of the mouth and advanced while pushing the tongue to the left. Take care not to damage any teeth or dental work. Advance the laryngoscope under direct vision without levering on the teeth; if the view is poor, pull the handle upwards in the direction of its axis. Keep the angle of the handle low. The tip of the curved Macintosh laryngoscope blade should follow the curve of the tongue until it rests in the vallecula; traction on the handle will lift the epiglottis and the larynx will come into view.

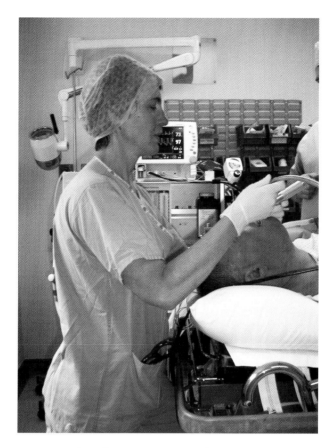

Figure 3.1 Laryngoscopy – anaesthetist standing.

Cormack and Lehane have classified the *laryngoscopic view* into four grades, illustrated in Figure 3.2. Laryngoscopic view depends very much on how far the epiglottis can be lifted in order to uncover the glottis. Grades I and II provide a full or partial view of the glottis, while in grades III and IV the epiglottis covers the glottis and therefore these are considered difficult. Only epiglottis is seen in grade III and no laryngeal structures in grade IV.

A further factor is a *straight line of vision*, i.e. alignment of the anterior edge of the incisors, the base of the tongue and the glottis. This depends on many factors but a substantial part of the work is to

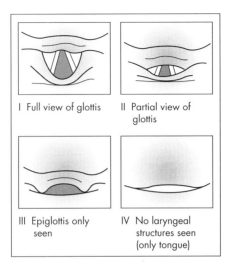

I Full view of glottis

II Partial view of glottis

III Epiglottis only seen

IV No laryngeal structures seen (only tongue)

Figure 3.2 Grades of laryngoscopy.

displace the tongue left and lift the lower jaw with traction, as described above. It is important for the anaesthetist to keep his/her back straight, as this improves the line of sight. Compensate with the lower part of your body if you are unable to alter the trolley height, instead of stooping (see Figure 3.3 for tips on improving the line of sight).

Difficult laryngoscopy and intubation is described in Chapter 11: The Difficult Airway.

Intubation
When the view is optimised, the anaesthetist grasps the tracheal tube with his/her right hand and passes it under direct vision between the vocal cords, to a *depth sufficient to prevent accidental extubation* (in cuffed tubes this is approximately 2–3 cm above the top end of the cuff; in pre-formed uncut tubes there should be a marker for depth of insertion) but not too far to prevent endobronchial intubation. Accidental *endobronchial intubation* tends to be on the right, as the left main bronchus is more deviated from midline, and leads to desaturation because of a resulting large shunt. When the tube is passed, the assistant inflates the cuff and the anaesthetist supports the tube until secured with a tie or a tape.

The assistant may help during laryngoscopy by retracting the corner of the mouth, providing laryngeal pressure, adjusting the pillow or passing extra equipment (bougie, Magill's forceps etc.) to the anaesthetist.

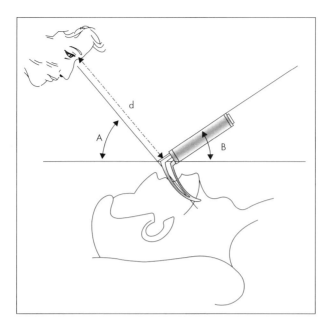

Figure 3.3 Angles at eye distance at laryngoscopy. A is the angle between the line of sight and the horizontal, B is the angle between the handle of the laryngoscope and the horizontal, and d is the distance between the heel of the laryngoscope and the eye. To optimise conditions, aim for a high angle A, low angle B and long distance d. (From Walker, J.D. Posture used by anaesthetists during laryngoscopy. British Journal of Anaesthesia, 2002, 89, 772–774.
© The Board of Management and Trustees of the British Journal of Anaesthesia. Reproduced by permission of Oxford University Press/British Journal of Anaesthesia.

Seeing the tube pass between the vocal cords is a good confirmation of its placement. However, in cases of difficulty the tube may only be seen to pass under the epiglottis. In all cases, confirm the position of the tube: *listen* over both lung fields in the axillae (breath sounds should be present on both sides equally) and over the stomach (air entry should be absent), *watch* the chest rise and fall, *observe* a typical capnographic trace – expiratory waves of equal height and with a plateau, reaching the same height >3 kPa of end-tidal CO_2 on repeated breaths (Figure 3.4a).

If there is a problem after intubation: high airway pressures, decreasing saturation, poor capnographic trace (Figure 3.4b), think **DOPE** (without thinking it, you would be one!).

ROUTINE INTUBATION

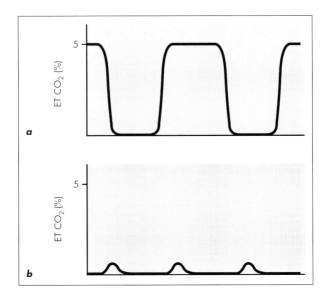

Figure 3.4 Capnographic trace with **a** tracheal intubation;
b oesophageal intubation.

The tube may be affected by:
- **D**isplacement – tube in the oesophagus or the right main bronchus
- **O**bstruction – by secretions or foreign body
- **P**neumothorax – suspect if high ventilation pressures were used; distinguish it from oesophageal and endobronchial intubation
- **E**quipment – any part of it may malfunction: get another device that is simple and quickly checked

Suspect *oesophageal intubation* in any of the following:
- Chest expansion is poor, hand ventilation difficult
- A guttural sound is heard during manual ventilation
- Capnographic trace shows small blips or no expired CO_2
- Oxygen saturation decreases
- Abnormal breath sounds/no breath sounds heard on auscultation
- Inflated abdomen/abdominal size increasing – this may be a late sign

A combination of these signs should increase the index of suspicion.

In case of difficult laryngoscopy (grades III and IV) and subsequent doubt as to the tracheal tube placement, perform a second laryngoscopy and attempt passing a second tracheal tube into the trachea, whilst leaving the first tube in situ. Connect the second tube to the breathing circuit and ventilate with 100% oxygen. If intubation was successful, suction the stomach after passing a nasogastric tube through the first (oesophageal) tube. If second intubation was unsuccessful, remove the tubes and ventilate with alternative means (mask and airway or laryngeal mask airway (LMA)).

The *capnographic trace* is not 100% reliable as a tool to confirm tracheal tube placement. The trace will be poor or absent if there is a large leak around the tube, in cases of severe bronchospasm (air trapping) and during cardiopulmonary resuscitation. If there is a doubt about the tracheal tube placement in a patient with severe bronchospasm, none of the tests relying on lung ventilation will be reliable. Confirmation must then be done by other means, i.e. visual – by direct laryngoscopy with the tube in situ. If unable to visualise the glottis, try pressing the tracheal tube backwards against the hard palate during laryngoscopy – this may bring the larynx into view. Transillumination with a light hand may also help with the diagnosis.

If unable to confirm the tracheal tube placement and saturations are decreasing, it is preferable to remove the tube and ventilate with alternative means [mask and airway or LMA and if necessary, surgical airway (see Chapter 11: The Difficult Airway)].

> **Remember:** Patients do not die of difficult laryngoscopy but they do die or get brain damaged from hypoxia. Saturations less than 60–70% lasting longer than 3 min would be expected to produce some detrimental effects. Take action to improve saturation before then.

Summary
1. Optimise conditions (equipment, staff, patient).
2. If in doubt, take it out!
3. Oxygenate, oxygenate, oxygenate.

Bibliography
Roberts JT. *Clinical Management of the Airway*. WB Saunders, 1994.
Walker JD. Posture used by anaesthetists during laryngoscopy. *BJA* 2002; 89(5): 772–774.

ROUTINE INTUBATION

Chapter 4

Abdominal Surgery

Andrew Taylor

Abdominal surgery covers a large range of procedures from ruptured abdominal aortic aneurysms to skin lesions. Some procedures can be done under local anaesthesia (e.g. local infiltration, spinal, epidural etc.). This chapter will discuss the conduct general anaesthesia. The airway required and the technique of achieving airway control will depend on the following factors:

• Type of operation
• Risk of regurgitation
• Post-operative plan (e.g. ventilate on intensive therapy unit (ITU))
• Duration of operation
• Need for paralysis and intermittent positive pressure ventilation (IPPV)

Type of operation
The most common abdominal operations are:

• Appendicectomy
• Bowel obstruction or perforation
• Abdominal trauma
• Hernias
• Laparoscopic procedures
• Gastrointestinal bleeds

Appendicectomy/bowel perforation/bowel obstruction/abdominal trauma
These operations have been grouped together because they all fall into the category of 'an acute abdomen'. An acute abdomen is any condition causing abdominal pain, requiring surgical intervention.

• Assume that patients requiring these emergency procedures have a full stomach, even if they have been 'nil by mouth' for more than 6 h.
• These operations will all need muscle relaxation to gain access to the peritoneal cavity and IPPV will be needed.

It is therefore necessary to rapidly achieve a definitive airway that will protect the trachea from soiling. These patients are intubated with a tracheal tube using a rapid sequence intubation (RSI), see following pages.

Non-obstructed hernia (inguinal/femoral/umbilical etc.)
These elective cases do not present the same risk of aspiration as the previous emergency cases. The condition itself does not necessitate the need for a RSI, but if the patient has other predictive risk factors for regurgitation (see below), then a RSI is indicated.

Assuming no regurgitation risk factors, this is a situation when discussion with the surgeon is necessary. Some surgeons will want the patient paralysed and ventilated as 'there is less straining in the muscles'. Some will prefer the patient to be self-ventilating, as 'I want the tissues to be in the positions they will naturally adopt'. If the patient is thin, has no other risks of aspiration and the surgeon is happy for them to be self-ventilating then a laryngeal mask airway (LMA) is adequate. If the surgeon requires muscle relaxation then it is safer to insert a tracheal tube.

Gastrointestinal bleeds

These patients present several difficulties and usually require the efforts of two anaesthetists and many assistants. As the patient has a 'full stomach', they are at risk of aspiration and anaesthesia should be induced with a RSI and tracheal intubation.

If the patient is persistently vomiting blood, he/she will not be able to lie flat for the duration of pre-oxygenation. One solution is to prepare for anaesthesia in the left lateral position, including pre-oxygenation. After anaesthesia is induced and cricoid pressure is in place, then assistants can help to turn the patient into the supine position. It may be necessary to have two working suction units in order to provide a clear view of the airway for intubation.

Aggressive fluid resuscitation should be employed with crystalloid or colloid in the first instance, then blood products when available. The dose of induction agents required is reduced in hypovolaemic patients.

Laparoscopic procedures

The limits of laparoscopic surgery are expanding rapidly. The list of procedures that can be carried out laparoscopically include hernias, cholecystectomies, appendices, hemicolectomies, Nissen's fundoplications, sterilisations as well as diagnostic laparoscopies. Laparoscopic procedures usually involve creating a pneumoperitoneum, i.e. inflating the peritoneal cavity with carbon dioxide, thus increasing the intra-abdominal pressure. This increase in pressure will reduce the efficacy of the lower oesophageal sphincter, increasing the chances of stomach content regurgitation. The increased pressure will also push up on the diaphragm, compressing the lungs, reducing pulmonary compliance and thus increasing the airway pressure for IPPV. Furthermore, some gynaecological procedures will require the Trendelenburg position to allow the bowel to fall away from the site of operation. For these reasons it is safer to insert a tracheal tube for laparoscopic surgery.

Laparoscopic Nissen's fundoplication is a procedure that is carried out to cure severe gastric reflux. It should be obvious that these patients are at risk of regurgitation and aspiration so anaesthesia should be induced with a RSI. It should be noted that even after the procedure, full cure may not be achieved and such patients presenting for further surgery are at risk of aspiration.

Risk of regurgitation

When awake, laryngeal reflexes protect the trachea from being soiled. The reflex action triggers cough and produces expulsion of any foreign material. When anaesthetised, this reflex is abolished. Aspiration of stomach contents into the airways can cause significant morbidity and mortality. Patients with an increased risk of regurgitation and aspiration include:

1. The *acute abdomen*. Any intra-abdominal pathology that causes abdominal pain/stasis/obstruction will lead to an increased risk of regurgitation. Patients with small bowel obstruction may have several litres of faeculent fluid sequestered in their stomach and small bowel.

2. Patients with an *incompetent lower oesophageal sphincter*. Patients with reflux or a hiatus hernia have a leaky sphincter, which may not prevent stomach contents passively entering the oesophagus. It is thought that nasogastric tubes, by passing through the sphincter, make it incompetent. (As a nasogastric tube would be passed in cases of bowel obstruction or vomiting, the risk of reflux existed a priori.)

3. Patients with *achalasia* of the oesophagus have a stenotic narrowed sphincter, which prevents swallowed food entering the stomach. Food pooling in the oesophagus then occurs.

4. Patients who have a *high intra-abdominal pressure* (e.g. obesity, pregnancy). If the pressure in the abdomen exceeds the pressure of the lower oesophageal sphincter, the stomach contents will be pushed through into the oesophagus. In addition, gastric emptying into the duodenum will be delayed. Some of the hormones released in pregnancy relax smooth muscle, reducing the competency of the lower oesophageal sphincter.

5. Patients who are *vomiting*.

6. Patients with a *full stomach*. Clear fluids should have left the stomach by 2 h, milk and food by 6 h.

7. Patients taking *drugs that slow gastric motility* (e.g. opiates, alcohol, tricyclic anti-depressants).

8. Patients with *trauma* that occurred soon after food intake.

Rapid sequence induction/intubation

RSI is a method of induction of anaesthesia where anaesthesia is induced after pre-oxygenation and airway protected from aspiration by a fixed sequence of events. The aim is to achieve rapid airway control and protection from aspiration as soon as anaesthesia is induced. Note the following points.

Preparation

- Explain to the patient what you are about to do.

- Explain specifically about pre-oxygenation and that they will feel some pressure on the front of their throat to prevent them being sick or regurgitating while anaesthetised.

- Only undertake RSI with the help of a trained anaesthetic assistant.

ABDOMINAL SURGERY

43

- Attach appropriate monitoring, minimum of non-invasive blood pressure (NIBP), ECG, pulse oximetry and capnography.
- Check if bed/trolley can be rapidly tilted head down.
- Check all necessary drugs that are drawn up, including suxamethonium and atropine, labelled and at hand.
- Ensure full resuscitation equipment available.
- Ensure 'good size' vascular access.
- Position the patient's head in the 'sniffing the morning air' position (flexion at the lower cervical vertebrae and extension at the atlanto-occipital joint) and adjust pillows as necessary.
- Place functioning suction/Yankauer catheter under pillow on right hand side.
- Pre-oxygenate for three full minutes with the patient taking standard breaths. This is the length of time required for the nitrogen in the lungs to be washed out and replaced with oxygen, creating the longest duration of time with apnoea for intubation before oxygen saturation starts decreasing.

Induction of anaesthesia
- Induce anaesthesia with a calculated dose of induction agent, given as a rapid bolus.
- No opiates are given at this stage, as they will prolong the duration of apnoea. The exception may be a patient with ischaemic heart disease.
- The assistant prevents passive regurgitation by using the Sellick's manoeuvre of cricoid pressure (Figure 4.1). This is achieved by pressing on the cricoid cartilage with the thumb and index finger with a force of 20 N (newtons) at the beginning of induction, increasing to 30 N when consciousness is lost. This pressure occludes the oesophagus behind the cricoid cartilage. The anaesthetic assistant should practise the force required regularly on training scales (a force of 10 N corresponds approximately to a weight of 1 kg): the aim is to develop a force corresponding to a weight of 2–4 kg (Figure 4.2).
- Achieve rapid muscle paralysis using a measured dose of depolarising muscle relaxant (suxamethonium 1.5 mg/kg). *Do not hand ventilate at this stage!*
- After fasciculations have subsided, perform laryngoscopy and intubate the trachea with a cuffed tube.
- The assistant should inflate the cuff with a pre-determined amount of air.
- Check the position of the tracheal tube by:
  - Watching both sides of the chest rise and fall.
  - Listening to both sides of the chest for air entry and the stomach for absence of air entry.
  - Observing at least six breaths of carbon dioxide during exhalation on the capnography trace.

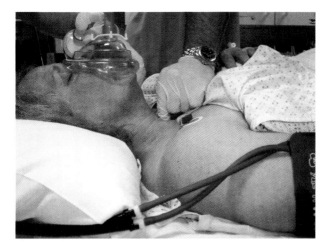

Figure 4.1 Application of cricoid pressure.

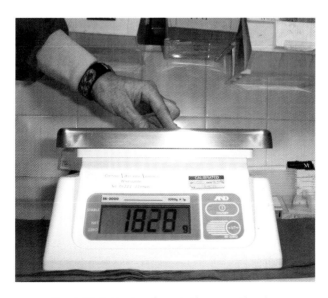

Figure 4.2 Training to perform cricoid pressure with scales.

ABDOMINAL SURGERY

- Listen for a leak around the cuff of the tracheal tube – add additional air as needed.
- The assistant should release the cricoid pressure only when clearly instructed to do so by the anaesthetist. This removes any misunderstandings that could lead to soiling of the trachea.
- If intubation is unsuccessful on the first attempt, then follow the failed intubation drill.

Regurgitation is a passive process that can occur when anaesthetised. Vomiting, however, is an active process and cannot occur when fully anaesthetised. If a patient starts to vomit when cricoid pressure is in place (indicating insufficient anaesthesia for application of cricoid pressure), cricoid pressure should be removed, as there is a risk of oesophageal rupture. The bed is tilted head-down and any vomitus is suctioned.

Extubation
It must be remembered that the patient is also at risk of tracheal aspiration at the end of a case when the tracheal tube has been removed.

- At the end of the procedure, the patient is placed in the *left lateral position*.
- *Muscle paralysis is fully reversed* (patients are able to open their eyes and lift their head off the pillow for 5 s; there should be no 'fade' or 'post-tetanic facilitation' on peripheral nerve stimulation).
- The patient should be:
  – *Breathing spontaneously* with breaths of appropriate tidal volumes.
  – *Breathing 100% oxygen*.
  – *Awake*, such that s/he can obey commands and demonstrate reversal of muscle paralysis.
- The tracheal tube is removed when the patient is effectively able to remove it by him/herself. This is the best way to be sure that the protective laryngeal reflexes have returned and the patient is able to protect their own airway.

Summary
- If the patient is at risk of aspiration then a rapid sequence induction should be considered.
- Procedures involving a breach of the peritoneum will require muscle paralysis, intubation of the trachea and ventilation. Muscle paralysis should be maintained up to the point of closure of peritoneum and muscle layer.
- 'If you consider a RSI or unsure then you should do it'.

Bibliography
Sellick BA. Cricoid pressure to prevent regurgitation of stomach contents during induction of anaesthesia. *Lancet* 1961; 2: 404–406.

Chapter 5
Trauma and Burns
Andrew Taylor

Since the introduction of advanced trauma life support (ATLS), the importance of rapid airway management and ventilation control has become paramount in a patient with multiple injuries. Doctors treating a trauma casualty should start their assessment by identifying and treating the injuries that will kill the patient quickest. Unidentified and *untreated problems with the airway will kill* before breathing problems, which kills before circulation problems. Therefore the order of the examination to be followed is:

- **A** – Airway
- **B** – Breathing
- **C** – Circulation
- **D** – Disability
- **E** – Exposure/Environment

It should be emphasised that when receiving any trauma or burns patient, the first consideration should be to assess and deal with any injuries to the airway and breathing, in that order. If the problem is identified, assessment is interrupted and the problem is treated until resolved.

Causes of airway embarrassment in trauma or burns
- Intrinsic: tongue, oedema, blood, dentures, food, vomit, other foreign bodies
- Extrinsic: fractures, haematomas, head and neck positioning

Causes of ventilation problems
Nervous system
- Respiratory centre injury
- CNS depressant drugs
- Spinal cord injuries

Musculoskeletal system
- Diaphragm injuries
- Rib fractures/flail chest
- Restriction to chest expansion by burns

Other
- Haemothorax
- Pneumothorax
- Drugs

Preparation
Preparation for trauma patients can be divided into long-term and short-term. Long-term planning will include hospital locations, ambulance service provision, accident and emergency departments, trauma

team staffing and training etc. Short-term preparation includes what should be done when advance warning has been received that a trauma patient is expected.

Trauma patients arriving at a hospital should be received in a dedicated resuscitation area that is equipped with the appropriate equipment to deal with the immediate management of their injuries. Check the equipment available while waiting for the arrival of the casualty.

- Facilities to supply supplemental *oxygen* to spontaneously breathing patients (piped or wall supplied oxygen, trauma mask with rebreathing bag).
- *Airway adjuncts* available to assist airway maintenance in the comatose or semi-comatose breathing patient (oropharyngeal and nasopharyngeal airways).
- Advanced airway equipment and equipment to aid *tracheal intubation* in a patient who is difficult to intubate (equipment for tracheal intubation, laryngeal mask airway (LMA)).
- Equipment to remove foreign bodies from the airway (Yankauer suckers, *suction* catheters for aspirating down nasopharyngeal airways or down tracheal tubes, Magill's forceps for removing solid material).
- Equipment for developing a *surgical airway* (cricothyroid membrane puncture and jet ventilation, tracheostomy).
- *Ventilation* equipment: Ideally a fully stocked anaesthetic machine (end-tidal CO_2 monitoring, self-inflating bag, portable ventilator and monitoring).
- Equipment specific to the details of the injuries that are expected, e.g. anaesthetic *drugs* for rapid sequence induction (RSI) of anaesthesia if a patient with a head injury and low Glasgow coma scale (GCS) is expected or *chest drain* equipment if a pneumothorax/haemothorax is suspected.

Burns
Thermal injury can take many forms. It can be the result of explosions, flames, smoke, steam and dry heat. The extent of the damage will depend on:
- Degree of heat
- Duration of thermal injury
- Injury occurring indoors or outside

The exact mechanism of the thermal injury is therefore important in predicting the likely pathology and hence the type of airway intervention required. The following examples aim to illustrate this:

1. *A patient who has thrown petrol onto a bonfire and received flash burns to their face in the open air would have sustained injuries to their face, lips etc.*

but protective reflexes would have spared the lower airway. As it would have been a thermal injury of short duration, the depth of injury and so the amount of oedema will be less, so tracheal intubation may not necessarily be required for reasons of airway obstruction.

2. A casualty who has been recovered unconscious from prolonged exposure inside a burning building is more likely to have both upper and lower respiratory tract damage. The injury will be as a result of direct heat as well as smoke inhalation. The potential for life threatening airway oedema and complete upper airway obstruction is high, while oedema of the fragile epithelium of the lower respiratory tract will reduce its ability to efficiently pass oxygen to the blood. This patient is more likely to require early tracheal intubation and ventilation to prevent catastrophic airway obstruction and hypoxaemia.

Problems with airway management in trauma patients

Airway management can be more difficult when faced with a patient in the emergency department than in the relative calmness of an anaesthetic room. The ability to deal with these situations is learnt with experience and senior help should be present to assist if difficulties arise.

The following factors complicate airway management in the emergency department:

- Because of potential cervical spine instability, the patient's neck movements may be restricted to prevent spinal cord damage (see below).
- The patient may have a full stomach.
- Inability to perform a complete airway assessment if the patient is semi-conscious.
- Unfamiliar surroundings and staff, different equipment or the lack of it. Limited space around patient, especially at the head end.
- 'Adrenaline factor' in staff.
- Airway trauma will distort the normal anatomy and blood in the airway will reduce the normal visibility, while partial airway obstruction will reduce the efficiency of pre-oxygenation.
- Undisclosed injuries, e.g. a simple pneumothorax that will become a tension pneumothorax when positive pressure ventilation is started.
- Unco-operative patients (alcohol, head injuries etc).

Airway with cervical spine control

All trauma patients must be assumed to have a cervical spine injury until proved otherwise. This means that the cervical spine must be maintained in a *neutral position* to prevent causing damage to the cervical cord. Before equipment becomes available you should hold

TRAUMA AND BURNS

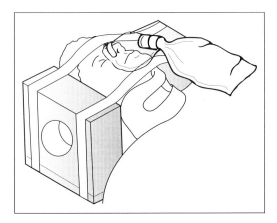

Figure 5.1 Patient with hard collar and head box (Redrawn with permission from Hodgetts T, Deane S, Gunning K. *Trauma Rules*. BMJ Books, 1997).

the head to prevent neck movement. The standard equipment to protect the cervical spine consists of:

- A *hard collar* around the neck restricting atlanto-occipital joint flexion and extension,
- *Sand bags or head box* next to the head to prevent lateral flexion and rotation, and
- *Straps* across the forehead and the chin to prevent neck flexion. See Figure 5.1.

Although protection of the cervical spine from further damage is important it should be remembered that airway obstruction and resulting hypoxia would kill before a spinal injury. For this reason, if the patient's airway is being compromised by stabilising the cervical spine, then the *airway* should *take priority*. There is no point in dying from hypoxia with an intact cervical spine!

If, for instance, a patient is vomiting, they will be turned on their side rapidly. The strapping should be released and the patient is allowed to turn on the side him/herself (a conscious patient will protect their cervical spine from serious injury). Unconscious patients by definition will not vomit but may regurgitate. If turning on the side is necessary, this should be done by 'log-rolling' in a controlled fashion, unless the airway is compromised, when it must be done promptly.

The signs of an *obstructed airway* are:

- Stridor, gurgling noise in throat or no inspiratory noise

- Tachypnoea
- Cyanosis
- See-sawing of chest and abdomen
- Use of accessory muscles of respiration
- Nasal flaring
- Absence of water vapour in the facemask on expiration

The presence of any of these signs would indicate that the airway is not patent. If the mouth is inspected, any foreign bodies or vomit can be seen and the tongue checked to ensure it has not been pushed back. Every patient should be treated as though they have an unstable cervical spine until you have proved otherwise. The manoeuvres 'head tilt' and 'chin lift' could both cause further injury to the spinal cord if the spine has been damaged. In trauma patients, the '*jaw thrust*' manoeuvre is used to pull the mandible forward thus pulling the tongue away from the posterior pharyngeal wall. This can be done without flexing or extending the neck.

Oropharyngeal and nasopharyngeal airways can be used as adjuncts to create a better airway. *Do not use a nasopharyngeal airway in a head injury* for fear of penetrating trauma through the base of the skull. Actively look for signs of airway obstruction and assign a member of staff for *continuous monitoring* of breathing.

Breathing with supplemental oxygen
If the patient is breathing spontaneously, place a trauma mask with a full reservoir bag connected to 10–15 l/min of oxygen over their face. Rapidly and systematically examine the respiratory system in trauma patients:
- *Inspection*
  - Count the respiratory rate. Look for equal chest movement on both sides. Look for any obvious chest wall deformities, e.g. flail segments.
- *Palpation*
  - Feel the trachea to assess whether it is deviated to either side. Palpate the chest for pain or fractures and feel for chest wall expansion.
- *Percussion*
  - Percuss both lungs from top to bottom to listen for any dullness (indicating blood) or hyper-resonance (indicating a pneumothorax).
- *Auscultation*
  - Listen to both lungs in the apexes, mid zones and bases to hear unequal air entry, added sounds or absence of breath sounds.

A *pneumothorax* occurs when air is trapped between the lung and the chest wall. They are termed 'simple' when the air can enter and leave

TRAUMA AND BURNS

the space or 'tension' when the air enters but does not leave, so the pressure in the chest rises and the lungs and heart become compressed. These are medical emergencies. The signs of a pneumothorax are:

• Reduced air entry on that side.
• Reduced chest expansion on that side.
• Deviation of the trachea away from the pneumothorax.
• Hyper-resonance to percussion on that side.

The immediate life-saving management of a tension pneumothorax is to decrease the intrathoracic pressure and 'let the air out'. To do this, *needle thoracocentesis* is performed. A large-bore (14 gauge) needle is inserted into the thorax on the side of the pneumothorax in the second intercostal space in the mid-clavicular line. This should be met with a hiss as the air inside is released under pressure. The cannula is left in situ and as the definitive management, a chest drain can then be inserted.

Why do patients with a pneumothorax need a chest drain before intubation?

Any patient with fractured ribs, pneumothorax, haemothorax or flail chest should have a chest drain inserted before being intubated and ventilated if at all possible. Patients in extremis may require intubation first, but emergency decompression will be required straight away.

When we breathe by ourselves, we suck air into our lungs by creating negative pressure in our chest. If the visceral pleura surrounding the lungs has been punctured, some of this air will pass into the pleural space. When intubated and ventilated, air enters the lung by positive pressure, i.e. air is blown in instead of being sucked in. This increased pressure in the lung will enable more air to pass into the pleural space, increasing the size of a pneumothorax more rapidly. A *simple pneumothorax* could be converted into a *tension pneumothorax*.

Tracheal intubation in the emergency department

Trauma casualties arriving in the emergency department are unlikely to have an empty stomach. Tracheal intubation, if required, will need to be carried out with the least risk of gastric content aspiration possible. This means using RSI (see Chapter 4: Abdominal Surgery), awake fibreoptic intubation (a specialist technique not described here) or a surgical airway. For reasons of skill, time and equipment, RSI is most commonly used. If the patient's cervical spine has been immobilised with a hard collar, tracheal intubation will be more difficult, as you will be unable to extend the head and flex the neck. In addition, the hard collar, if fitted correctly, will limit the patient's mouth opening. To overcome these problems, the straps and sandbags can be removed during RSI and tracheal intubation if the cervical spine is held

TRAUMA AND BURNS

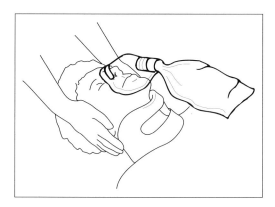

Figure 5.2 Manual in-line stabilisation from the head end (Redrawn with permission from Hodgetts T, Deane S, Gunning K. *Trauma Rules*. BMJ Books, 1997).

immobilised by an assistant. The hard collar, or at least the front portion of it, has to be removed in order to enable the anaesthetist to open the mouth and to apply cricoid pressure if applicable. The *manual in line stabilisation* can be done by two methods:

1. The assistant crouches at the head end of the bed, next to the person responsible for intubating the trachea and holds each side of the head and neck (Figure 5.2).
2. The assistant stands next to the patients' chest facing the patient and holding the head and neck.

Surgical airway in the emergency department

The need for a surgical airway can be semi-elective, if the patient is still able to maintain oxygenation and ventilation, or it can be an emergency procedure when the airway is no longer patent. Surgical airways can be achieved with local anaesthesia and reassurance in a co-operative patient. This avoids the risk of losing the airway under sedation or general anaesthesia.

There are three types of surgical airway.

1. Crico-thyroid puncture or cricothyroidotomy

A wide-bore needle or a custom made cannula of a 4 mm internal diameter is inserted through the crico-thyroid membrane to gain access to the trachea. Oxygen can then be insufflated into the respiratory tree. This method is the fastest but does not achieve a 'definitive airway'.

2. Percutaneous dilational tracheostomy (PDT)

This is the procedure used on many intensive care units to perform tracheostomies, so it is familiar to many anaesthetists. The trachea is located by aspirating air through a needle and syringe. A guidewire is inserted through the needle over which dilational bougies are 'rail roaded' to make a sufficient lumen for a tracheostomy tube to pass. Newer systems have a one-step tapered dilator. This procedure is usually done in patients who are already intubated and expected to need prolonged intubation.

3. Formal surgical tracheostomy

This procedure is usually carried out by surgeons and requires more extensive dissection to visualise the trachea directly. It can be done under local anaesthetic.

Summary

- Airway and breathing problems will kill trauma patients before other injuries.

- All trauma patients have a cervical spine injury until proved otherwise.

- Patients with pneumothoraces should have chest drains inserted before intubation and positive pressure ventilation.

Bibliography

Advanced Trauma Life Support Manual, Chicago. Amercian College of Surgeons, 1997.

Chapter 6

The Paediatric Airway

Priti Dalal

This chapter will focus on:

- Anatomical differences between the paediatric and the adult airway
- Paediatric airway equipment
- The technique of airway management in children

Before discussing the paediatric airway, it is important to understand the following terms:

Term	Age
Pre-mature	<37 weeks gestational age
Post-mature	>42 weeks gestational age
Neonate	First 28 days or <44 weeks post-conception
Infant	1 month to 1 year of age
Child	1 year to adolescence

Anatomical differences between the paediatric and the adult airway

There are several differences between the paediatric and the adult airway that can make airway management more difficult in children. The airway of older children may be similar to adults. However, in cases of neonates and infants, there are several important differences that one needs to bear in mind.

1. Neonates have a large head relative to the body causing difficulty during intubation as the head may wobble during laryngoscopy.

2. Infants are obligatory nose breathers.

3. The large tongue and small mouth make laryngoscopy more difficult.

4. The epiglottis is large and floppy and protrudes into the pharynx.

5. The larynx is at a higher level (C3–C4) compared to adults (C4–C6).

6. The larynx is at a more acute angle, making intubation more difficult.

7. The vocal cords are angled more forwards and downwards as a result of which the tip of the tube has a tendency to touch the anterior aspect of the larynx during intubation.

8. The narrowest part of the infant's airway up to 8 years of age is at the level of the cricoid cartilage. The adult larynx is cylindrical compared to the funnel shaped larynx in the infant. It is therefore possible to pass the tube through the larynx and then it is difficult to negotiate it through the subglottic region.

9. The infant's trachea is deviated downwards and posteriorly and is shorter.

THE PAEDIATRIC AIRWAY

10. The ribs are horizontal, leading to inefficient movement of the rib cage during respiration.

11. The intercostal muscles are not well developed and the breathing is mainly diaphragmatic.

12. The diaphragm is prone to fatigue as it has fewer type 1 fibres.

13. The surfactant that lines the alveoli, preventing airway collapse, only develops after 32 weeks of gestation. The pre-mature baby therefore may be more prone to respiratory distress.

The following table highlights the problems that can be expected during management of the paediatric airway:

Airway	Problem	Management
Large head and occiput	Positioning during mask ventilation or intubation Overextension may cause airway obstruction	Steady the head during laryngoscopy, head in neutral or slightly flexed position Avoid hyperextension
Obligate nose breathers	Airway obstruction	Use of oropharyngeal airway
Small mouth, large tongue, Large tonsils	Visualisation during laryngoscopy difficult	Proper technique Correct size and type of blade
Large and floppy epiglottis	Laryngoscopy difficult	Better visualisation if the tip of the laryngoscope blade includes the epiglottis
Larynx at higher level (C3–C4)	Airway obstruction	Straight or less curved blades are more useful for laryngoscopy
Vocal cords angled forwards and downwards	Tip of the tube abuts against the anterior aspect of the larynx	Careful intubation
Narrowest part at the level of the cricoid cartilage	Damage to the tracheal mucosa	Select uncuffed tube, correct fit means allowing an audible leak at inflation pressures of 20 cm water
Shorter tracheal length	Endobronchial intubation common	Correct length of the tube, auscultation to confirm bilateral air entry

Respiratory physiology

In addition to the anatomical differences, there are several differences in the respiratory physiology from the adult that can affect airway management in the neonate and the infant:

	Neonate (3 kg)	Adult
Oxygen consumption (ml/kg/min)	6–8	3.5
Carbon dioxide production (ml/kg/min)	6	3
Tidal volume (ml/kg)	6	6
Respiratory rate (per minute)	32–35	12–16
Vital capacity (ml/kg)	35	70
Functional residual capacity (FRC) ml/kg	30	35

The *increased oxygen consumption* and *carbon dioxide production* make the neonate prone to hypoxia. Hence, even small periods of apnoea during difficult airway management may not be well tolerated. The reduced FRC and increased closing volume result in early closure of the airway during tidal ventilation. The work of breathing is also increased due to the increased resistance offered by the narrow air passages. It is for these reasons that many anaesthetists prefer to electively ventilate the patient.

Airway diameter
According to the Hagen-Poiseuille formula, in the case of laminar flow, the flow through a tube (Q) is directly proportional to the pressure drop across the tube (P) and the radius (r) raised to the power of 4 and inversely proportional to the viscosity (η) of the fluid and the length of the tube (l):

$$Q = \frac{P \cdot \pi r^4}{8 \eta l}$$

This has dual significance:
1. A small reduction in the diameter of the airway due to oedema will markedly reduce the flow and increase airway resistance, increasing the work of breathing.
2. Selection of a proper size tracheal tube is important as too tight a fit can lead to subglottic oedema.

Neonatal and infant anaesthesia is a specialist field for the experienced anaesthetist. However, junior trainees may be called to paediatric cardiac arrest or trauma situations and therefore knowledge of paediatric airway management is vital.

Paediatric airway equipment
Breathing systems
In case of older children weighing more than 15–20 kg, an adult breathing system can be used. However, in children weighing less than

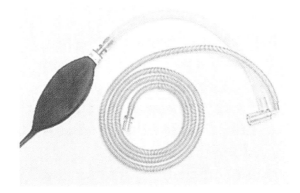

Figure 6.1 Ayre's T-piece with Jackson-Rees modification (Reproduced with permission from Al Shaikh B, Stacey S. *Essentials of Anaesthetic Equipment*, 2nd edn. Elsevier Science Ltd, 2002).

15–20 kg, due to the reasons mentioned previously in this chapter, a special breathing system to meet their physiological requirements must be used.

An ideal breathing system in small children should have the following characteristics:

- Minimal dead space
- No valves or a single low resistance valve
- Minimal gas turbulence and flow resistance
- Light weight
- Easy to use

The Jackson-Rees modification of the *Ayre's T-piece* (Figure 6.1) is the most commonly used breathing system in paediatric anaesthetic practice. This consists of three limbs. One limb connects to the fresh gas flow via long tubing. The second limb connects to the mask or tracheal tube at the patient end. This limb is kept as short as possible to reduce the dead space. The third limb is the expiratory limb. This is attached to a long section of corrugated tubing, at the end of which lies an open tail-ended reservoir bag. The bag is the Jackson-Rees modification and is designed so as to reduce air dilution during inspiration, and enable assisted ventilation with continuous positive airway pressure (CPAP).

Masks
Paediatric masks are so designed as to allow a good fit with minimal dead space. Many different types of masks are available. Facemasks

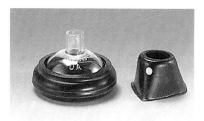

Figure 6.2 Clear plastic and Rendell-Baker mask (Reproduced with permission from Al Shaikh B, Stacey S. *Essentials of Anaesthetic Equipment*, 2nd edn. Elsevier Science Ltd, 2002).

made of clear plastic have the advantage in that any condensation vapour during expiration and vomitus can be clearly seen. The Rendell-Baker masks have the advantage of having a smaller dead space (Figure 6.2).

Oropharyngeal airway
The most commonly used is the Guedel airway. A range of sizes is available (see Chapter 7: Airway Management Without Intubation). The size is chosen to approximate the distance between the corner of the mouth and the angle of the mandible.

Laryngoscopes
A straight blade laryngoscope (Figure 6.3) gives a better exposure in infants as the glottis may be viewed by lifting the epiglottis. It also occupies less space and thereby gives more room for intubation. Laryngoscope blades that are less curved may also be used (i.e. the standard Macintosh). The handles of the laryngoscopes are of a smaller diameter.

Tracheal tube
Uncuffed tubes are used in children upto size 6. Various types are available. Single use tubes are now used routinely. The universal (oral/nasal) uncuffed tube, cut to size, and the pre-formed RAE tube (see Chapter 10: Head and Neck, Maxillo-Facial Surgery, ENT and Neurosurgery) are most commonly used. The Cole pattern tube has a specially designed shoulder so as to prevent endobronchial intubation.

Selecting the *correct size*, i.e. internal diameter of the tracheal tube is important. The most commonly used formula is: (age ÷ 4) + 4. An

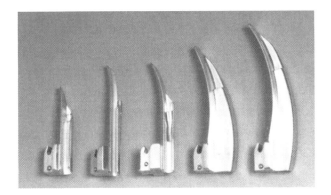

Figure 6.3 Paediatric laryngoscope blades of various sizes (left), shown for comparison with two adult size blades. (Reproduced with permission from Hutton P, Cooper GM, James FM and Butterworth JF. *Fundamental Principles and Practice of Anaesthesia*, Martin Dunitz, 2002.)

important point to remember is that there should be an audible leak with inspiratory pressures of 20–25 cm of water. If the tube fit is too tight, there is the possibility of tracheal mucosal oedema leading to airway obstruction following extubation. It is also important to have the correct *length* of the tube; otherwise there is a chance of endobronchial intubation. The commonly used formula for length in centimeters is: (age ÷ 2) + 12. At the age of 20 this comes to 22 cm – the adult length.

Age of the patient	Internal diameter of the tube (mm)
Pre-term	2.5
At birth	3.0–3.5
6 months	4.0
1 year	4.5
Over 2 year	Age/4 + 4

Intubation technique

In the past, awake intubation was performed routinely in neonates. This practice is no longer recommended as it is difficult to intubate a strong, fighting infant, generating a massive stress response. Awake intubation may increase the incidence of periventricular haemorrhage in pre-mature infants or those with coagulopathy. For these reasons, a controlled induction is now preferred. Neonatal anaesthesia is a specialist field but the anaesthetic senior house officer (SHO) may come across cases of neonatal resuscitation.

The following sequence may be used for induction and intubation in children:

1. A thorough *history* is taken and the airway examined on the ward. In young children presenting with upper airway problems/surgery, anti-cholinergic pre-medication may be of value. This can be given orally except in the neonate or very young infant. The parents should be informed about the conduct of the anaesthetic and the likely problems (unco-operation, smelly vapour, failure of topical anaesthetic cream etc.).

2. All the *apparatus*, anaesthetic machine and patient details must be checked.

3. Make sure that suction equipment is present.

4. The *airway equipment* consists of a range of suitable-sized masks, airways, laryngeal mask airways (LMAs) and tracheal tubes of the appropriate size, connectors and the breathing system. Make sure that at least a size smaller and a size larger tracheal tube is also available.

5. Although *pre-oxygenation* is ideal and is used in the adults, a child on arrival to the induction room may be crying, spluttering and unco-operative unless a pre-medication has already been given. The child may need to be gently coaxed and cajoled into an inhalational induction, with parental help if the parents are present. Skilled assistance is invaluable. The combination of oxygen-sevoflurane is commonly used. An *intravenous induction* (Figure 6.4) may be possible in older children. Propofol is licensed for use in children above the age of three. A muscle relaxant may or may not be used for

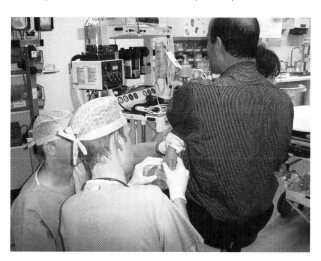

Figure 6.4 Paediatric intravenous induction (parent present).

intubation. Suxamethonium is used in paediatric anaesthesia in the UK at a dose of 1 mg/kg.

6. Make sure the child is *adequately anaesthetised*, as children are prone to laryngeal spasm, vomiting and aspiration during the lighter planes of anaesthesia.

7. Remember to start *monitoring* as soon as the child is asleep if this has not been possible before the anaesthetic induction. In addition, bear in mind that monitoring can never replace vigilance and clinical judgement.

8. Correct *positioning* of the patient is important. Overextension may cause airway obstruction or irritate the larynx causing a laryngeal spasm.

9. An *intravenous access* can be achieved once the child is asleep and the airway is under control if this has not been possible prior to induction.

10. Use an *oropharyngeal airway* if necessary, especially in an overweight child with a large tongue.

11. Gentle positive pressure breaths must be delivered for two reasons – to *avoid gastric insufflation* of air thereby causing regurgitation and aspiration, and to avoid barotrauma.

12. Depending on the age and size of the child, a straight or a slightly curved laryngoscope may be used. For a right-handed person holding the *laryngoscope* in the left hand, position the head, open the mouth of the patient and taking care of the lips, carefully introduce the laryngoscope blade. Carefully lift the handle at the same time moving the tongue away onto the left side exposing the larynx. If it is difficult to visualise, gently adjust the tip of the blade. Slight external pressure on the cricoid by an assistant may help to visualise the larynx. Then, the tracheal tube may be passed gently so that it does not hit the anterior commissure of the larynx but slides through into the trachea. The *tracheal tube* should then be connected to the breathing system. Correct *placement must be checked* by visualisation of chest expansion, auscultation of the chest and the epigastrium and using the end-tidal carbon dioxide monitor. It is also important to avoid endobronchial intubation. With uncuffed tubes, check for an *audible leak* on gentle inflation. If no leak is heard, replace tube with one half a size smaller. To compensate for the leak, use relatively high gas flow for intermittent positive pressure ventilation.

If there is any doubt regarding placement of the tracheal tube then one should be prepared to take the tube out and ventilate with a facemask. Always call for *senior help* when there are problems with the management of the airway.

Causes of difficult airway in children may be classified as:

1. Congenital
2. Acquired

The congenital syndromes, which may make airway management difficult in children, are shown in the table:

Congenital problem/syndrome	Airway problem
Down	Large tongue, small mouth, large tonsils, atlanto-axial instability
Goldenhar	Unilateral mandibular hypoplasia, cervical spine abnormality
Klippel-Feil	Cervical vertebral fusion
Pierre-Robin	Micrognathia, glossoptosis, cleft palate
Treacher-Collins	Micrognathia, cleft palate, mandibulo-facial dysostoses
Turner	Difficult intubation
Cleft palate	Problems with laryngoscopy

The acquired conditions in children where airway problems may be expected are:
- Trauma and burns
- Infection
  - epiglottitis, laryngotracheobronchitis
- Neoplastic
  - laryngeal papillomatosis
- Others
  - foreign body, post-intubation laryngeal oedema

Management of the difficult airway in children requires special skills and expertise and such patients are best managed in specialist paediatric centres.

Consent and co-operation to undergo anaesthesia
When handling children, bear in mind the level of understanding and co-operation that can be expected. Neonates, infants and toddlers up to the age of 3–4 cannot be expected to understand the need for surgery and anaesthesia. For the very young neonate, a careful explanation to the parents and parental absence during the induction is preferred. For children aged 1–4, induction of anaesthesia is best turned into a game (blowing up balloons, hugging parent, snuggling up etc.). Remember that if the child resists gas inhalation during induction, it will also lighten anaesthesia. Resistance may often be seen in stage II of Guedel's classification (excitement). Warn the parents beforehand – you may liken the situation to the loss of inhibition in moderate alcohol excess – and explain the need for some restraint at this stage (in order to allow anaesthesia to continue).

THE PAEDIATRIC AIRWAY

Older children who have an understanding of what they are about to undergo require an explanation. The induction can still be a game (playing pilots, laughing gas) but if the child resists the gentlest of persuasion or restraint, induction of anaesthesia cannot proceed until both the parents' and child's co-operation is obtained.

Summary

1. Children are not small adults. They desaturate quickly.

2. Use uncuffed tracheal tubes up to size 6 and ensure that there is a leak around the tube.

3. Make a plan but be prepared to adapt your technique to individual circumstances.

Bibliography

Cote CJ. Pediatric anesthesia; in Miller RD (ed): *Anesthesia*, 5th edn. Churchill Livingstone, Volume 2, Chapter 59, p 2088.

Moyle JTB, Davey A. Equipment for paediatric anaesthesia; in: *Ward's Anaesthetic Equipment*, 4th edn. WB Saunders, Chapter 14, pp 231–243.

Stoelting R, Dierdorf S. Diseases common to the pediatric patient; in: *Anesthesia and Co-existing Disease*, 3rd edn. Churchill Livingstone, Chapter 32, pp 579–583.

Chapter 7

Airway Management Without Intubation

*Priti Dalal and
Andrew Taylor*

The first part of this chapter describes how the airway is maintained without airway adjuncts and with the aid of supraglottic devices. Methods of delivering supplemental oxygen are discussed in the second part of this chapter.

Airway management without intubation (AMWI) is an important skill that must be mastered by the medical staff.

It may be carried out:
- As a part of primary airway management prior to emergency or elective intubation.
- When intubation equipment or intubation skills are unavailable, e.g. on the wards or out of hospital scenarios.
- When intubation is difficult.
- When the patient has a partially obstructed airway.
- As a part of a general anaesthetic.

The upper airway has a rigid wall supported by the vertebrae posteriorly and a collapsible anterior wall formed by the tongue and the epiglottis anteriorly (Figure 7.1). The anterior wall obstructs the airway if there is a loss of muscle tone (unconsciousness, paralysis), or if the bulk of the soft tissue is increased (oedema, abscess, tumour).

AMWI may consist of the use of one or more of the following:
- Triple manoeuvre
- Facemasks
- Oropharyngeal airway
- Nasopharyngeal airway
- Laryngeal mask/oesophagotracheal Combitube/airway management device

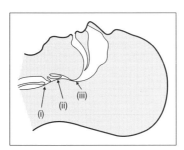

Figure 7.1 The airway may be obstructed by the larynx (i), epiglottis (ii) and/or tongue (iii) pressing on the posterior part of the pharyngeal wall.

The triple manoeuvre

This classically consists of:

- Head tilt
- Chin lift
- Jaw thrust

The aim of this manoeuvre is to establish patency of the collapsed airway so as to allow the passage of air for gas exchange.

Head tilt
The operator gently places his/her hands around the patient's forehead so as to achieve upper cervical extension.

Chin lift
The operator places the tips of his/her index and the middle finger underneath the patient's chin, over the bone so as to gently lift it up.

Jaw thrust (Figure 7.2)
The operator brings the mandible forward by placing the index and other fingers of both his/her hands behind the angle of the mandible, applying steady upwards and forward pressure to lift the mandible. The thumbs are used to displace the chin downwards and open the mouth.

The head tilt and chin lift is avoided in patients with suspected head or cervical spine injury.

Facemasks

Facemasks are designed so as to fit snugly over the patient's mouth and nose. The purpose of the facemask is to deliver oxygen, plus/minus

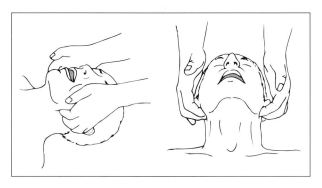

Figure 7.2 Jaw thrust.

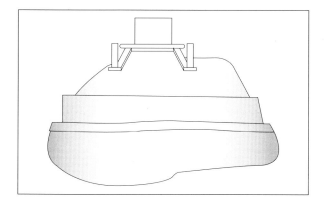

Figure 7.3 Anaesthetic facemask (Redrawn with permission from Davey AJ, Moyle JTB, Ward CS (ed.): *Ward's Anaesthetic Equipment*, 4th edn. WB Saunders, 1997).

anaesthetic gases from the breathing system to the patient. A mask has a mount, a body and a peripheral seal. The mount connects to the breathing system. The body and seal may be made of black rubber or disposable plastic. The transparent plastic mask has the advantage that it allows the detection of gas exchange in the form of condensed vapour, and also of vomit. The inner volume of the facemask constitutes the dead space. This may become significant in paediatric patients. The peripheral seal comes in contact with the face: it may have a cushion (which may be filled with air or a soft mouldable material), or a flange (Figure 7.3).

Facemasks are used:

1. To deliver anaesthetic gases during spontaneous or controlled ventilation
2. During resuscitation

The facemask may be held either with one hand or two hands.

One hand technique
The thumb and the index finger are placed on the body of the mask on the opposite side of the mount. These fingers are used to push the mask downwards to give an airtight seal. The distal phalanges of the ring and the middle fingers are used to lift up the jaw and extend the neck. The tip of the fifth finger is placed at the angle of the mandible and is used to lift up the jaw. The other hand may then be free to squeeze the reservoir bag to deliver positive pressure breaths.

Two hand method
In this technique, both the thumbs are placed on either side of the mount and the index fingers are used to support the body of the facemask. The rest of the fingers are used to lift up the jaw on either side and extend the neck. An assistant has to squeeze the bag if assisted ventilation is required.

Complications
1. Improper fit may cause gas leak, ineffective ventilation and inadequate anaesthesia.
2. Too large a mask may cause trauma to the eyes.

The oropharyngeal airway (Figure 7.4)
When properly sited, the oropharyngeal airway lifts up the posterior part of the tongue and the epiglottis from the posterior pharyngeal wall, allowing the patient to breathe through the lumen of this device. It has a curvature to conform to the shape of the tongue. It has three parts: the flanges, the bite portion and the curved body. The oral end has a flange that acts as a guard to limit the depth of insertion. This leads to the flat bite portion followed by the curved body that follows the curvature of the tongue. The device has a lumen to maintain airway patency. In addition, it also allows passage of a suction catheter to facilitate suctioning and clearing oropharyngeal secretions. When in use, the teeth of the patient rest against the bite portion. The pharyngeal end lies just above the epiglottis. There are different sizes available from 000, 00, 0, 1, 2, 3 and 4. They are colour-coded (Figure 7.5).

Indications
1. Airway obstruction in a spontaneously breathing patient with obtunded airway reflexes.
2. To facilitate intermittent positive pressure ventilation (IPPV) and oxygenation prior to intubation.

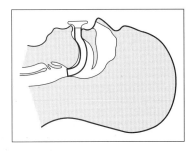

Figure 7.4 Oropharyngeal airway in use.

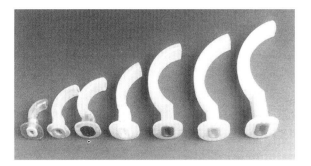

Figure 7.5 Guedel oropharyngeal airways in different sizes (Reprinted with permission from Davey AJ, Moyle JTB, Ward CS (ed.): *Ward's Anaesthetic Equipment*, 4th edn. WB Saunders, 1997).

Contraindications (relative)
1. Patients with very loose teeth and fragile dental work.
2. Inadequately anaesthetised patients.

Method of insertion
The correct size is chosen (the correct size for a patient is determined by the distance between the corner of the mouth and the tragus).

It is then lubricated and inserted with the curvature initially facing upwards and then rotated halfway through so as to follow the curvature of the tongue. In edentulous patients, it may also be inserted right from the outset with its curvature along the curvature of the tongue. Once inserted, it is very important to support the jaw to maintain patency of the airway.

Problems and complications
1. Incorrect size, if used, may not correct the airway obstruction.
2. The pharyngeal end of the device may stimulate coughing, retching and laryngospasm in a partially anaesthetised patient.
3. Damage to the teeth, dislodgement of caps or crowns may occur.

Nasopharyngeal airway (Figure 7.6)
This consists of a soft plastic, polyurethane or latex rubber tube that can be placed in the nasopharynx. It has nasal and pharyngeal ends and a curved tubular body. The pharyngeal end has a bevel to facilitate atraumatic insertion of this device. The nasal end has a flange with safety pin to prevent the airway slipping into the nasopharynx. There are various sizes available, described by the internal diameter.

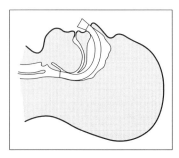

Figure 7.6 Nasopharyngeal airway.

Indications
1. Patient with limited mouth opening
2. Loose dentition
3. As an alternative to the oropharyngeal airway
4. To facilitate nasotracheal suctioning

Contraindications
1. Patients with bleeding diathesis
2. Maxillo-facial fractures
3. Basal skull fractures
4. Recent nasal surgery
5. History of epistaxis

Method of insertion
The correct size for the patient is chosen. The wider nostril is traditionally chosen, although it may bear little relationship to the internal size of the nasal passage. The airway is lubricated and the insertion takes place through the nares, passing along the floor of the nose (i.e. vertically down in a supine patient) and into the oropharynx until the tip lies just above the epiglottis.

Complications
1. Trauma – the nasal mucosa, the turbinate, adenoids
2. Bleeding

The laryngeal mask airway (LMA)
This device is used in an anaesthetised patient for maintaining the airway during both spontaneous and controlled ventilation. It is passed through the mouth until the distal end lies over the laryngeal inlet. It has a proximal end, a curved hollow tubular body and a distal end. The proximal end has a 15 mm male connection which can be attached to

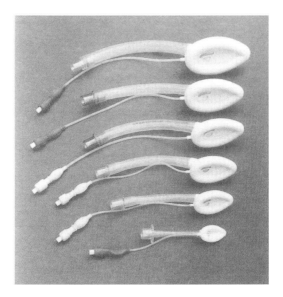

Figure 7.7 Laryngeal mask airway in sizes 1–5 (Reprinted with permission from Davey AJ, Moyle JTB, Ward CS (ed.): *Ward's Anaesthetic Equipment*, 4th edn. WB Saunders, 1997).

the breathing system. The distal end has an elliptically expanded cuff which, when inflated, positions the distal end of the tube snugly over the laryngeal inlet. The distal end of the tube is fenestrated with two thick strands to prevent the epiglottis from occluding its lumen. The cuff has a pilot tube with a pilot balloon and a self-sealing valve so that the cuff remains inflated when injected with air. It is made up of silicone rubber, can be sterilised by autoclaving and reused. The maximum amount of time it can be reused is 40 times, as recommended by the manufacturer. Disposable prototypes have now been developed. There are different sizes available (Figure 7.7):

Size	Patient type/ weight (kg)	Cuff inflation volume (ml)
1 Neonates, infants	Up to 5	Up to 4
11/2 Infants	5–10	Up to 7
2 Infants, children	10–20	Up to 10
21/2 Children	20–30	Up to 14
3 Paediatric	30–50	Up to 20
4 Adults	50–70	Up to 30
5 Adults	70–100	Up to 40
6 Large adults	Over 100	Up to 50

There is a longitudinal black line on the tubular conduit of the LMA for ease of positioning. When correctly placed, this line should lie dorsally and in the midline.

The reinforced LMA has a steel spiral incorporated in the wall of the tube to give it flexibility and at the same time prevent it from kinking. It is often used for oral, maxillo-facial and ENT surgery.

Indications
These can be classified as emergency or elective.

Emergency
• To secure the airway in a case of failed intubation
• A difficult intubation
• To buy time for another definitive form of airway

Elective
• It may replace the facemask to provide hands free anaesthetic.
• It may replace the tracheal tube in oral and maxillo-facial surgery.
• As aid to intubation – e.g. passing a bougie through the LMA and then railroading the tracheal tube over it, or passing a fibreoptic laryngoscope through the LMA and then passing the tracheal tube.

Contraindications
Where there is a risk of aspiration, such as:
• Patients with full stomach
• History of active reflux or a hiatus hernia
• Major surgery
• Morbidly obese patients
• Pregnancy (elective surgery from 16 weeks up to 48 h post delivery)

Method of insertion
There are several techniques that have been described for insertion of the LMA. The standard technique is described below:
1. Inflate the cuff up to 50% of its maximum volume and check for cuff leaks.
2. Deflate the cuff fully or partly and apply a lubricant jelly to lubricate the back of the cuff (i.e. the pharyngeal side).
3. Ensure that the patient is adequately anaesthetised.
4. Extend the patient's neck and stabilise the occiput so that the jaw falls open. The assistant may help by holding the patient's mouth open.
5. Grasp the LMA like a pen in the dominant hand and press the distal tip of the deflated LMA cuff against the hard palate using the index finger of the non-dominant hand to guide the tube over the back of the tongue and into the oropharynx.

6. Advance the LMA gently until characteristic resistance is felt as it engages the upper oesophageal sphincter.

7. The cuff is then gently inflated with air not exceeding the maximum recommended volume.

8. The LMA may 'float out' slightly with this manoeuvre as it tries to fit itself in the correct position.

9. The LMA is then connected to the breathing system.

10. Correct position is checked with gentle positive pressure breaths showing chest expansion, noticing the movements of the reservoir bag in a spontaneously breathing patient, auscultation and watching the end-tidal carbon dioxide trace. The black line on the tube of the LMA lies dorsally in the midline.

When correctly inserted, the distal end of the cuff lies immediately above the oesophageal sphincter with its tip resting in the inferior recess of the hypopharynx. Its sides face into the piriform fossa and the upper border rests against the base of the tongue. The LMA must be properly secured with a tape or a tie so as to avoid any displacement.

When the LMA is used for controlled ventilation, it is important to keep inflation pressures not greater than 20 cm of water, otherwise it may result in gastric insufflation.

There are other methods of insertion of the LMA. These include – holding it like a dart during insertion, use of a malleable introducer, inserting it like an oropharyngeal airway with the concave side facing upwards and then rotating it half way through the mouth and inserting while facing the patient, using the thumb to aid advancement.

Complications

1. Immediate – related to poor insertion technique
   - Trauma to the teeth, pharyngeal mucosa, anterior pillar, epiglottis, tonsils
   - Damage to the LMA cuff by sharp teeth
   - Retching, coughing and laryngospasm in a lightly anaesthetised patient

2. Delayed – related to prolonged use or high cuff inflation pressures
   - Pharyngeal mucosal oedema
   - Hypoglossal, glossopharyngeal nerve palsy
   - Sore throat – usually mild and short-lived
   - Dysphagia, dysphonia, hoarseness of voice
   - Displacement of the LMA during surgery
   - Aspiration of gastric contents or blood

Since its early days the LMA has developed into six different forms:

1. The *classic* LMA.
2. The *reinforced LMA-Flexible™*, a LMA with a flexible, wire reinforced shaft that can be bent but will not kink.
3. The *LMA®UNIQUE*, a single use, disposable LMA.
4. The *ilma®*, a LMA that comes with a cuffed silicone tracheal tube which will pass through the lumen of the LMA into the trachea.
5. The *LMA Pro-Seal®*, a LMA with an extra lumen to allow the passage of an oro-gastric tube into the stomach to reduce the risk of gastric content aspiration into the trachea.
6. The yellow non-metallic valve assembly for use in MRI units.

Other supraglottic devices

The range of supraglottic airways available is still changing. Besides the LMA the other options available are:

- Airway Management Device, AMD™, Nagor Ltd, Douglas, Isle of Man
- Combitube™, Tyco Healthcare Ltd, Gosport, UK (Figure 7.8)
- Cuffed Oropharyngeal Airway, COPA™, Tyco Healthcare Ltd, Gosport, UK
- Laryngeal Tube, LT®, VBM GmBH, Sulz, Germany (Figure 7.9)
- Pa$_x$™ oropharyngeal airway, Pa$_{xpress}$™, Vital Signs Ltd, Barnham, UK (Figure 7.10)

The COPA™ has recently stopped being produced and will soon be unavailable. New supraglottic airway devices are in the production

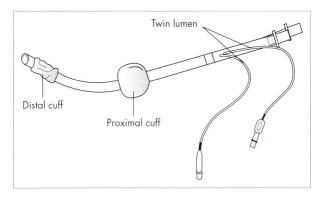

Twin lumen

Distal cuff

Proximal cuff

Figure 7.8 Combitube.

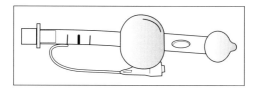

Figure 7.9 Laryngeal tube.

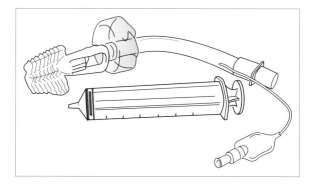

Figure 7.10 Pa$_{xpress}$.

stages at present and may well appear in general circulation in the near future. These include:

- Laryngeal Tube Sonda, LTS®, VBM GmBH
- Streamlined Liner of the Pharynx Airway, SLIPA™ SLIPAmed UK, London, UK
- Soft Seal Laryngeal Mask, Portex Ltd, Hythe, UK

The Combitube

The Combitube is a device originally produced in the USA, mentioned here for the sake of completeness. It is essentially a double-lumen tube, which can be introduced blindly over the tongue to provide ventilation irrespective of whether it is placed in the trachea or the oesophagus. It has a large proximal cuff designed to inflate in the hypopharynx. There is also a small distal cuff. The tracheal lumen has an open distal end, whereas the oesophageal lumen has several small side holes located between the two cuffs.

The device is introduced blindly and 95% of the time it enters the oesophagus. In this case the lungs are ventilated via the oesophageal lumen with the air/oxygen escaping via the side holes, which are in close proximity to or above the larynx. The closed end of the oesophageal lumen and the inflated proximal cuff prevent any gas leaking through the mouth. If the distal end is in the trachea, ventilation can be achieved through the distally open ended tracheal port.

It has the following disadvantages:

- Adequate mouth opening is required for its insertion
- It can cause trauma to oropharyngeal structures
- Risk of oesophageal rupture
- Ventilation of the wrong port (i.e. oesophagus) can cause oesophageal rupture and subcutaneous emphysema

It is used little in Britain because of unfamiliarity and the potential complications.

Oxygen supplementation

It may be necessary to give supplemental oxygen to an awake, spontaneously breathing patient in the anaesthetic room or in the operating room under the following circumstances:

- A patient who has had a regional or central neural blockade
- A patient who has had intravenous sedation
- While preparing for or attempting fibreoptic intubation

Oxygen supplementation can be achieved by using various devices. They may be classified as variable or fixed performance devices. The variable performance devices are nasal catheter, nasal prongs and a facemask (e.g. Hudson mask). These devices deliver a variable amount of inspired oxygen depending on the oxygen flow rate and the patient's inspiratory effort. The *fixed performance* devices, on the other hand, consist of a venturi device that can be attached to the facemask, LMA, tracheal or a tracheostomy tube entraining a known amount of air at a set oxygen flow rate. The fixed performance devices are used mainly on the ward or the high dependency units. For prolonged controlled oxygen administration, the venturi device is attached to a wide-bore tubing and the gas is warmed and humidified. Because the venturi no longer delivers controlled oxygen directly to the patient's face, the final concentration of oxygen delivered will again depend on the patient's minute ventilation, if it exceeds the volume of the system.

The following are the *variable performance devices* used in the induction or operating room.

Nasal cannula/nasal catheter
This consists of a foam padded catheter or a cannula which is inserted into one of the nostrils. The other end is connected to a tubing which

is connected to an oxygen source. This enriches the inhaled air with oxygen. It is best tolerated at low flow rates of up to 2 l/min. It is better tolerated than an oxygen mask which some patients may find suffocating.

Nasal prongs

This consists of plastic tubing with two small protrusions each of which fits into one nostril. The tubing is connected to an oxygen source at a flow rate of 2–3 l/min. The continuous flow of oxygen displaces the air, creating a reservoir of oxygen in the nasopharynx. The inspired oxygen concentration varies according to the oxygen flow rate and the patient's inspiratory effort.

Facemasks

These are clear plastic masks available in different sizes, connected via tubing to the oxygen source. Oxygen concentration delivered to the face depends on the oxygen flow rate and the minute volume. They can deliver inspired oxygen concentrations of 40–90% at flow rates of 3–15 l/min.

Summary

Supraglottic airways

- Are used for the majority of operations in the UK at the present time.

- Are useful to overcome airway obstruction, but do not protect the trachea from gastric content aspiration.

- Should be considered early to provide oxygen in the 'failed intubation' situation.

Bibliography

Al-Shaikh B, Stacey S. Tracheal and tracheostomy tubes and airways, masks; in: *Essentials of Anaesthetic Equipment*, 2nd edn. Churchill Livingstone, Chapters 5 and 6, pp 44–59.

Cook TM: Novel airway devices: Spoilt for choice? *Anaesthesia* 2003; 58: 107–110.

Moyle JTB, Davey A. Airway management devices; in: *Ward's Anaesthetic Equipment*, 4th edn. WB Saunders, Chapter 9, pp 139–147.

Moyle JTB, Davey A. Equipment for the inhalation of oxygen and entonox; in: *Ward's Anaesthetic Equipment*, 4th edn. WB Saunders, Chapter 10, pp 179–185.

Resuscitation Council (UK). Airway management and ventilation; in: *Advanced Life Support Course – Provider Manual*, 4th edn. Chapter 5, pp 31–38.

Valentine J, Stakes AF, Bellamy MC: Reflux during positive pressure ventilation through the laryngeal mask. *BJA* 1994; 73: 543–544.

AIRWAY MANAGEMENT WITHOUT INTUBATION

Chapter 8

Airway Management in Obstetrics

Sylva Dolenska

The obstetric patient may present for anaesthesia for planned or emergency obstetric procedures (Shirodkar suture, Caesarean section, manual removal of placenta), or emergency general surgical procedures (e.g. appendicectomy). Intubation may be required in some obstetric emergencies, e.g. eclampsia. Elective surgery is only carried out if it cannot wait until after delivery. Second trimester is relatively safe for administration of general anaesthesia, as organogenesis is completed and the risk of premature labour is low. If possible, procedures should be carried out under regional anaesthesia, when airway management is limited to administration of oxygen via facemask or nasal cannulae. However, even if regional anaesthesia is planned, the anaesthetist must fully assess the airway and be prepared for complications or failure of regional anaesthesia.

Physiological changes in pregnancy bring about important anatomical and physiological differences; these start gradually but become significant from about 16 weeks' gestation onwards.

The changes concerning airway management are:

- Stomach emptying is delayed and therefore there is an increased risk of aspiration of stomach contents even in a starved patient.
- Functional residual capacity (FRC) (and therefore oxygen reserve) is reduced and minute ventilation is increased; end-tidal pCO_2 is lower in pregnant subjects than in non-pregnant ones.
- Oxygen consumption is higher. Because of this and the reduced oxygen reserve, pregnant women desaturate more quickly than non-pregnant ones.

Towards term, there are a few more considerations:

- Work of breathing in a supine anaesthetised patient is increased because basal alveoli are collapsed at the end of expiration, the diaphragm is splinted and intra-abdominal pressure is increased.
- Enlarged breasts may make intubation difficult.
- The necessity for lateral tilt, in order to avoid aortocaval compression and hypotension, may make intubation difficult: cricoid pressure is usually applied in a perpendicular direction. With a left lateral tilt, this means that the larynx will be displaced towards the left.
- In pre-eclampsia and eclampsia, the larynx may be oedematous.

Assessment

In elective surgery, detailed assessment and preparations can be made. Systematic enquiry and examination along the lines suggested in Chapter 1: Airway Assessment, forms the basis of the assessment. Also ask about the course of the pregnancy, sickness, heartburn or reflux, breathing problems, heart disease and symptoms and signs of pre-eclampsia.

AIRWAY MANAGEMENT IN OBSTETRICS

Explain the need for rapid sequence induction if general anaesthesia is planned, what it involves and what risks it carries (see Chapter 4: Abdominal Surgery).

In an emergency situation, full history and assessment may not be possible, depending on the urgency of the surgical intervention or the medical condition. An apnoeic and/or hypoxic patient requires tracheal intubation and ventilation with 100% oxygen without delay. In a patient whose consciousness is obtunded, history may be obtained from relatives or staff caring for the patient. While making preparations to intubate, enquire about current cardiorespiratory status, medication, allergies and any previous difficulties with breathing during or after anaesthesia.

Pre-medication

Because most anaesthetic drugs reach the foetus, sedative pre-medication is withheld. From 16 weeks onwards, measures against acid aspiration have to be taken. Therefore prescribe an H_2 blocker (e.g. nizatidine 150 mg orally) and metoclopramide 10 mg, given at least 1 h pre-operatively, plus a non-particulate antacid (e.g. 30 ml of sodium citrate), given less than 30 min before induction. Ranitidine 50 mg i.v. is given if there is no time to give nizatidine orally.

Choice of airway device

A facemask with or without Guedel airway, or a laryngeal mask airway (LMA) may be used in non-obese pregnant women up to 16 weeks gestation, provided there is no history of heartburn or reflux. LMA may also be used in an emergency in the event of failed intubation (see Chapter 11: The Difficult Airway).

Rapid sequence induction and intubation of the trachea is the method of choice for airway management in anaesthetised patients above 16 weeks.

Conduct of general anaesthesia

Rapid sequence induction in pregnant women, and women up to 48 h after delivery

Because of diminished oxygen reserve and potential problems with the obstetric patient, the senior house officer (SHO) with less than a year's experience in anaesthesia should not anaesthetise this category of patients without direct supervision.

Use *left lateral tilt* (15°) or a *wedged position* after 16 weeks in singleton pregnancy (Figure 8.1), or 12 weeks in multiple pregnancy, to avoid aortocaval compression. If hair is tied at the back, loosen the hair band so that it does not preclude head positioning.

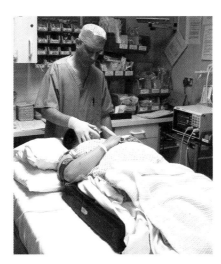

Figure 8.1 Left uterine displacement by a wedge.

Pre-oxygenate for a full 3 minutes using high flow oxygen and a well-fitting facemask. Use full *monitoring*, including capnography.

Prevention of *hypertensive response* to intubation is needed in hypertensive or pre-eclamptic women. Alfentanil 500 μg to 1 mg and/or labetalol 5–20 mg bolus are suitable (inform the paediatrician if using alfentanil).

All existing *intravenous induction* agents have been used in pregnancy. Thiopentone or propofol in a normovolaemic patient are given in a relatively generous dose, taking into account the increased metabolic rate (7 and 3 mg/kg, respectively). Etomidate should be reserved for the partly exsanguinated patient. It is emetogenic, suppresses the adrenal function in mother and foetus and causes superficial thrombophlebitis. Ketamine has been successfully used in Caesarean section. However, an antisialogogue may be needed with it. It may not be a suitable agent in a situation where bleeding is not controlled for fear of increasing the blood loss along with the increase in blood pressure.

Cricoid pressure is applied gradually during the induction of anaesthesia, so that when consciousness is lost, cricoid pressure is fully on. Cricoid pressure should be applied in the sagittal plane, i.e. perpendicular to the table (but not the floor), to avoid lateral displacement of the larynx. See Chapter 4: Abdominal Surgery, for full details of rapid sequence induction. The incidence of difficult intubation in obstetrics may be as high as 1 in 300 and incorrect application of cricoid pressure may be a contributing factor.

The *choice of neuromuscular blocking agent* has been a subject of debate. For the junior trainee, *suxamethonium* at a dose of 1.5 mg/kg is still the best choice. Pregnant women have less pronounced fasciculations and rarely have muscle pain after suxamethonium. The onset of muscle relaxation is fast but so is the offset. If difficulties are encountered at intubation, do not give a second dose of suxamethonium (second syringe of suxamethonium is often kept drawn up, to be used in case the contents of the first syringe is inadvertently spilled out or extravasating).

For the skilled intubator, high dose rocuronium has the advantage of fairly fast onset and medium duration of block. The longer duration of block is an advantage in failed laryngoscopy or intubation, provided ventilation can be maintained. It gives time to prepare alternative methods of intubation and avoids gagging, salivation and possibly hypoxia associated with the offset of neuromuscular block after an unsuccessful attempt with suxamethonium. Failure to ventilate after giving a non–depolarising muscular blocker would be disastrous; this, however, would be extremely unlikely in skilled hands, as the failed intubation in obstetrics is mainly due to operator or assistant's inexperience. With the exception of abnormal anatomy, morbid obesity or gross airway obstruction (e.g. in laryngeal oedema), hand ventilation can usually be achieved in the paralysed obstetric patient.

Conduct of intubation

Have a range of laryngoscopes, intubation aids and tracheal tubes ready.

After induction of general anaesthesia, application of cricoid pressure, and the onset of muscle relaxation, pass chosen laryngoscope (*short-handle* (Figure 8.2) is often the first choice) in usual manner and use an appropriate size tracheal tube (e.g. smaller tube in pre-eclampsia). Have a capnograph sampling tube connected to the breathing system filter. When the tracheal tube is passed, the assistant inflates the cuff and the anaesthetist stabilises the tube, connects the breathing system and gives several manual breaths of 100% oxygen. If the chest rises and falls, breath sounds are heard over the lung fields and capnographic trace indicates normal breaths (same size excursions reaching plateau), *tracheal intubation* is confirmed and cricoid pressure may be released. Nitrous oxide may then be added (50% or less for category 1 or 2 Caesarean sections, i.e. lifesaving or potentially threatening emergency and up to 66% for categories 3 or 4 – urgent but stable and elective procedures) and also a volatile agent to give at least one minimum alveolar concentration. It is important to start the *inhalational anaesthetic* at a sufficient dose after tracheal intubation is confirmed to avoid the

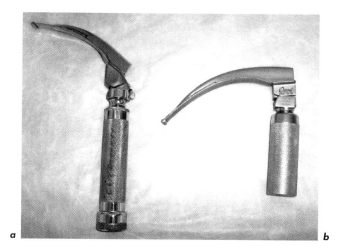

a *b*

Figure 8.2 **a** Polio blade; **b** Short-handled laryngoscope – alternatives in obstetric patients.

danger of awareness. This is particularly pertinent in the obstetric patient because opioids are often withheld until delivery, to avoid neonatal respiratory depression. The tube is fixed in position (usually with a tie), artificial mechanical ventilation may start, and a non-depolarising neuromuscular blocker may be given after three minutes.

Ventilate to end-tidal CO_2 around 4 kPa (see notes above on physiological changes in pregnancy).

If unable to pass the tube at first attempt, try to optimise the head position and use necessary aids (Magill's forceps, bougie). If still not successful and neuromuscular block is wearing off or oxygen saturation starts decreasing, follow the failed intubation algorithm (see Chapter 11: The Difficult Airway). Usual *mistakes*, which make a potentially easy intubation difficult, include:

• Insufficient *pre-oxygenation* – make sure that the oxygen (and oxygen only!) is turned on fully and the breathing system is intact and connected to the anaesthetic machine!

• Insufficient dose of *intravenous induction* agent (coughing, gagging on application of cricoid pressure) – administer more agent and instruct assistant to reduce the cricoid pressure temporarily. Be sure that the cannula is still intravenous.

• Too much *cricoid pressure* – often seen in less experienced assistants. If you can see the epiglottis but cannot lift it, or the anatomy is distorted, ask the assistant to reduce the cricoid pressure. If you can see the vocal cords but cannot pass the tube, use a smaller size tube and ask assistant to reduce the pressure. Vomiting is unlikely in a fully anaesthetised patient. Passive regurgitation may occur, that is why you have suction at the ready!

- Cricoid pressure is applied not perpendicular to the neck – see notes above.
- Cricoid pressure applied above or below the cricoid cartilage – check before induction whether the assistant knows where to apply the pressure. If pressure still applied in the wrong place, ask assistant to remove it completely and guide his/her fingers to the cricoid cartilage.

Extubation

The risk of *aspiration* of stomach contents persists after delivery for 48 h. Passing a large-bore orogastric tube and emptying the stomach before extubation has been advocated. Such measures should certainly be employed in patients who had a history of recent food intake. Perform oropharyngeal suction before extubation.

Extubate after reversing the neuromuscular block and a sufficient period of nitrous oxide washout. Position patient on her left side and check that laryngeal reflexes have returned, muscle power is near normal, gas exchange is good and the patient is sufficiently awake to wish to remove the tube.

If difficulty was encountered at intubation, anticipate difficulty at extubation – senior staff must be present. Perform *cuff leak test* in pre-eclampsia (see also Chapter 12: Extubation and Post-Operative Airway Management).

Summary

1. In obstetric anaesthesia and resuscitation, two lives depend on maternal oxygen delivery.
2. Risk of regurgitation and aspiration exists from 16 weeks onwards up to 48 h post delivery – use rapid sequence induction.
3. In case of difficult airway, oxygenation takes precedence over protection against aspiration.

Bibliography

Yentis S, Brighouse D, May A. *Analgesia, Anaesthesia & Pregnancy: A Practical Guide*. Saunders, 2000.

Chapter 9

Surgery in the Prone Position

Andrew Taylor

Surgery in the prone position (Figure 9.1) means the patient will be positioned face down on the operating table. It is easy to see that this will cause some problems to the anaesthetist, who is used to having full access to the patient's face and mouth throughout the surgical procedure. It is important to keep in mind that the anaesthetist needs to be able to maintain oxygenation, ventilation and airway protection while the patient is prone as well as when they are being turned prone.

Airway assessment

The pre-operative airway assessment of a patient about to undergo surgery in the prone position does not differ from the standard airway assessment (see Chapter 1: Airway Assessment). These patients will require tracheal intubation, so a plan needs to be decided on how best to achieve this.

Operations that require the patient to be prone include:

- Spinal surgery
- Pilonidal sinus
- Posterior chest wall surgery
- Other orthopaedic and neurosurgical procedures
- Percutaneous nephrolithotomy

While in neurosurgery and spinal surgery the need for the prone position is not questioned, other procedures can mostly be done in the

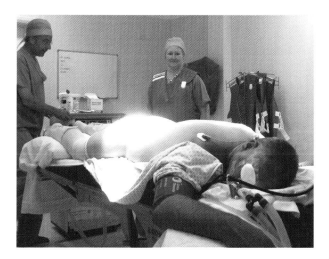

Figure 9.1 A patient lying prone.

semiprone or lateral position, which allows better access to the airway and poses less of a challenge to the circulation.

Problems associated with prone surgery:
- Airway
    - Airway device moving while patient is turned prone
    - Airway lost while prone
    - How to secure the tracheal tube
    - How to prevent tracheal tube occlusion
    - Changing airway while prone
- Breathing
    - Pressure on abdomen splinting diaphragm
    - Pressure on chest splinting ribs
- Circulation
    - Haemodynamic challenge of prone position
- Other
    - Pressure points and peripheral nerve protection
    - Venous access
    - Eye protection
    - Arm positioning
    - Head and neck positioning
    - Monitoring and defibrillation while prone
    - Prevention of fall
    - Safety of staff

Conduct of anaesthesia
The patient should be checked in to the anaesthetic room and standard monitoring equipment attached. Anaesthesia is induced in the supine position in the same manner as in any other procedure. Ensure you have good-flowing, large-bore venous access established and after intubation apply eye protection. This should take the form of protective eye ointment on the conjunctiva; eyelids taped closed and then padding is applied to the eyelids.

Which airway?
The safest option is to insert a *reinforced tracheal tube* (Figure 9.2). The reinforcement is a coil of metal, like a spring, that runs the length of the tube in the wall. This makes it harder to occlude the lumen of the tube when it is bent or kinked. Normal tracheal tubes will kink or bend at the point they leave the mouth, creating the risk of airway obstruction. As the reinforced tubes are designed to be more flexible and curve rather than kink, they are made of a less stiff type of plastic. This means that they are more floppy, which may in turn make them

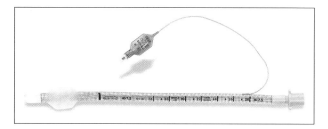

Figure 9.2 The Portex reinforced tracheal tube (Courtesy of Portex Ltd).

harder to insert. To solve this problem, a semi-rigid stylet can be inserted inside the reinforced tube before use. This will enable the tube to be pre-formed into a shape that will ease intubation. Laryngoscopy and intubation can then proceed as usual. Reinforced tubes do not protect the airway from occluding if the patient bites them, as the coil will deform. The metal coil precludes reinforced tubes being cut to length like standard tracheal tubes, so the anaesthetist should be aware of the chance of endobronchial intubation. Prone ventilation can be achieved with a laryngeal mask airway (LMA) but it is not recommended.

How to fix tracheal tube (Figure 9.3)

After intubation, the patient is going to be rolled onto their front, slid onto the operating table and may have their neck rotated, all before the operation starts. This process will then be reversed at the end of the procedure. You want to be as certain as possible that the tracheal tube will not become displaced. To do this, an oropharyngeal (Guedel) airway is commonly used as a bite block. The tracheal tube can then be stuck in place. Using two lengths of 2.5 cm wide elastoplast 20 cm long, secure the tube to the correct length at the teeth. Then, for added security, two lengths of 10 cm elastoplast, one cut as trousers and the other as underpants can be passed over the top to secure the whole assembly. The tube needs to be secured to a large area of skin because secretions escape from the mouth during surgery and could cause loosening of tapes and extubation. Patients with beards present a problem as the elastoplast does not stick well around the tube. Tie and tape may be better, or you could ask the patient to shave before the operation.

Cautious anaesthetists also insert a *throat pack*, as an additional protection against tube displacement and additional protection in case of cuff seal malfunction.

How to turn prone

There are many ways to turn an anaesthetised patient prone. It is important that a plan, previously agreed by all those responsible for the

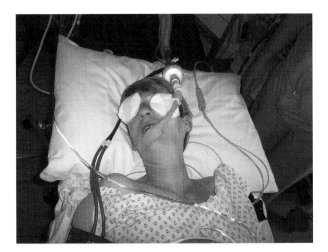

Figure 9.3 Equipment for securing tracheal tube.

turn is used, so as to improve patient and staff safety. The anaesthetist has overall responsibility for the position change, at the same time paying attention to maintenance anaesthesia, ventilation, oxygenation and support of the head.

Move the patient's bed alongside the operating table and apply and *check breaks*. Position two strong assistants on both sides of the patient (Figure 9.4). Position pillows on the operating table to support the chest and the pelvis, leaving the abdomen free to move with respiration. Alternatively a *Montreal mattress* (Figure 9.5) can be used. The assistants who are next to the operating table should stretch out both their arms across the table ready to receive the patient. Before turning the patient, the lungs should be ventilated with *100% oxygen plus vapour* for a few minutes. There are two schools of thought regarding what to do with the *monitoring* when turning a patient prone. The first is to remove all monitoring with the possible exception of a pulse oximeter, so as to avoid getting wires trapped, pulled or damaged during the turn. This means that the patient is unmonitored for the duration of the turn. The second option is to keep all monitoring in place and functioning, including invasive pressure monitoring if in use, so as to ensure patient safety. This means that meticulous care needs to be taken of all attachments during the turn, to protect both the patient and the equipment from damage.

On the anaesthetist's command turn-off the ventilator and *disconnect tracheal tube* from ventilator tubing. The two assistants next to the

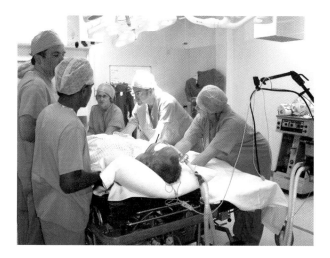

Figure 9.4 Position of helpers to turn prone.

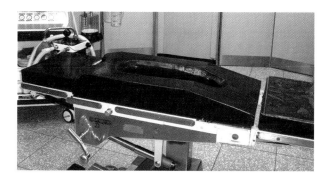

Figure 9.5 Montreal mattress.

patient's bed can then roll the patient onto the other assistants' arms. An alternative to this would be to turn the patient prone on the bed and transfer them prone onto the operating table. You must make sure that the head and neck stay *in alignment* with the rest of the body during the turn. After the turn is completed, position the head rotated to the side, provided the patient has no neck problems. Alternatively, use a horseshoe-shaped padded support. Re-connect ventilator tubing and *re-commence ventilation*. Attach monitoring, if previously removed. Remember that the position of ECG electrodes may need to be altered at this stage to achieve the best signal quality. Check if the eye on the dependent side is free from pressure. Arms should be kept by the side or put at right angles on 'vein board', and adequately protected from pressure or too much abduction.

After moving the patient and before he/she is covered with drapes, it is important to *confirm the position of the tube*. Check if both sides of the chest are visibly moving. Check if you can hear good air entry on both sides of the chest and there is no air leak from the mouth. Finally, check whether the tube is at the same length at the teeth as it was before the positioning and check if there is a good CO_2 trace on the capnograph. A decrease in oxygen saturation at this point may be an indication of endobronchial intubation due to the changed head position.

Ventilation
Ventilating in the prone position alters the chest wall compliance. The ribs are fixed to the spine posteriorly but are relatively free anteriorly at the sternum. This means that when ventilating in the *supine* position, the ribcage is able to spring open anteriorly, favouring ventilation of the anterior lung segments, while perfusion of the lung, which is gravity dependent, will favour the posterior lung segments. When the patient is positioned prone, the anterior part of the ribcage is splinted by its contact with the operating table. This should increase the ventilation of the dependent part of the chest, where perfusion is maximal, thus reducing ventilation-perfusion mismatch. When prone, chest expansion is achieved by the 'bucket handle' movement of the lateral ribcage moving superiorly and the diaphragm moving inferiorly. Poor support may make ventilation difficult and adjustment of the supports may be necessary.

Wake-up test
After spinal surgery, it was a previous practice for the surgeon to ask for a 'wake-up test'. This was to ensure that the spinal cord was still functioning after the spine had been corrected of any mal-alignment and was carried out in the prone position. Muscle relaxation was reversed and the depth of anaesthesia was allowed to lighten *sufficiently to be able to test the motor and sensory pathway*. This test has become somewhat redundant now with the increased use of spinal evoked potentials, but is included here for historical interest and completeness.

Extubation
When the surgery has been finished, it is safest to turn the patient back into the supine position before you start to reverse muscle paralysis or lighten anaesthesia. When the patient is supine, start your usual extubation process, e.g. check for the need to reverse paralysis if necessary. When self-ventilating, extubate awake or deep as required. Be aware that patients who have been prone are more likely to have

a lot of secretions in and around their oropharynx, so have suction equipment to hand. Remember to remove the throat pack if one was used. Insert an oropharyngeal airway to prevent the patient biting the armoured tube. If muscle relaxation was mainly achieved by deep inhalational anaesthesia, reversal of neuromuscular block is fairly easily achievable. For further information on the management of extubation, see Chapter 12: Extubation and Post-Operative Airway Management.

Summary
- A cuffed reinforced tracheal tube is the airway management device of choice for prone surgery.
- A reinforced tube is more flexible and may need a stylet to aid insertion.
- Reinforced tubes do not get cut to length.
- After moving any patient you should recheck the position of the tube.
- Pay attention to protection of eyes and pressure points.

SURGERY IN THE PRONE POSITION

Chapter 10

Head and Neck, Maxillo-Facial Surgery, ENT and Neurosurgery

Andrew Taylor

This chapter aims to highlight the potential difficulties in airway management that surgery in these specialities produces. Firstly we discuss the choice of airway devices available, the pros and cons of their use, and how the anatomical site of the operation affects the choice of airway device. Finally, the main topics of concern for the anaesthetist in the practice of anaesthesia for these specialities are dealt with in brief. It is beyond the scope of this book to describe fully airway management for all the procedures in these specialities.

Airway devices and equipment (Figures 10.1–10.3)
A list of abbreviations is provided at the end of this chapter.

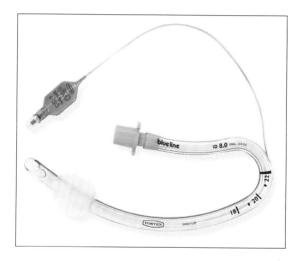

Figure 10.1 The Portex RAE tube – south-facing (Courtesy of Portex Ltd).

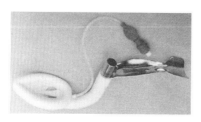

Figure 10.2 Intubating laryngeal mask airway.

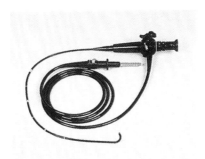

Figure 10.3 Fibreoptic laryngoscope.

Options for airway control — standard

	Advantages	Disadvantages
COETT	Best airway	Failure, trauma, connectors in the way
RAE tube (fig. 10.1)	Standard laryngoscopy, allows access to palate, pharynx	Pre-formed – fixed length, compression by gag
Armoured ETT	Protects tube from kinking if surgeons move head	Not cut to length, may need stylet to insert
Microlaryngeal ETT	Allows surgeon to visualise vocal folds	Insertion with Magill's forceps, compression
Nasal ETT	Blind insertion or laryngoscopy, oral cavity free, better tolerated by semi-conscious patient	Avoid in # base of skull, may cause nose to bleed
Laryngeal mask airway (LMA) – standard, flexible, intubating (fig. 10.2)	Easy to insert	No cuff in trachea, may reflect vomitus into larynx

Options for airway control — specialist

	Advantages	Disadvantages
Tracheostomy	Post-op ventilation, good supraglottic access, reduced dead space	Skilled personnel, invasive, traumatic, haemorrhage, displacement
Jet ventilation (Cricothyroid puncture or via Ravussin needle and rigid scope)	Can maintain oxygenation in cases of difficult intubation and ventilation, cricothyroid stab inserted under local anaesthesia	Invasive, personnel experience, equipment availability, no cuff in trachea, risk of aspiration, barotrauma

The following table outlines the methods available to insert the airway devices along with the advantages and disadvantages.

	Advantages	Disadvantages
Blind	Avoids laryngoscopy	Trauma, bleeding, often need to move neck to insert
Laryngoscope	Direct vision	Trauma, hypertensive response, education
Fibreoptic laryngoscope (fig. 10.3)	Awake option, fixed or stabilised neck	Expensive, experience, secretions and blood in airway
Retrograde	Another option	Equipment available, lack of experience

Site of surgery

Anatomically, these types of surgery can be split into six groups:

• Cranium

• Nose and sinuses

• Maxilla

• Mandible

• Pharynx

• Larynx

Each slightly alters the problems faced by the anaesthetist in airway management.

Obviously, some extensive surgical procedures will encompass several of these anatomical areas. The following table gives examples of procedures involved in each anatomical area and some of the potential problems encountered.

	Examples of procedures	Airway problems
Cranium	Burr holes, craniotomy	Airway under drapes throughout surgical procedure; sometimes prone position
Nose and sinuses	BAWO, septoplasty, rhinoplasty	High potential for blood to soil airway, 'coroners clot', left pack
Maxilla	Osteotomy, dental work	Airway compression, jaw wired post-op, blood soiling airway, left pack, swelling

HEAD AND NECK, MAXILLO-FACIAL SURGERY, ENT AND NEUROSURGERY

Table (continued)

	Examples of procedures	Airway problems
Mandible	Osteotomy, fractures, cysts, dental work	Same as for maxilla
Pharynx	EUA, tonsils, adenoids, tumours	Airway compression, blood soiling
Larynx	EUA, biopsies, laryngectomy, cysts	Complete airway obstruction, difficult intubation, airway compression or dislodgement

Shared airway

The most important point to emphasise in shared airway surgery is that of the *team approach*. The anaesthetist must allow the surgeons access to the operative field to allow the surgery to take place, while at the same time the surgeon must allow the anaesthetist to maintain oxygenation and ventilation.

It is essential that the anaesthetist and the surgeon involved in the case have discussed exactly what the procedure will involve and have formulated a joint plan to each other's satisfaction. The anaesthetist's main priority is to maintain oxygenation and ventilation at all times, while providing the best possible surgical access. Maintenance of general anaesthesia can be separated from airway management by the use of total intravenous anaesthesia (TIVA). If the surgeon requires access to the nose and/or pharynx, then a *RAE tube* that sits discretely on the tongue should ensure adequate access. *LMAs* are used increasingly in nasal surgery, with or without the use of an oropharyngeal pack. If the case involves visualisation of the vocal cords, then a 5 mm *microlaryngoscopy tube* allows the visualisation of most of the vocal cords. For complete surgical access to the cords, it is possible to induce anaesthesia and ventilate with a LMA until the surgeon is ready for laryngoscopy. The LMA is then withdrawn and the larynx ventilated with *jet ventilation* via a Ravussin needle attached to the laryngoscope.

Airway obstruction

Airway obstruction can be *complete* when no gases are able to pass from the anaesthetic system into the lungs or *partial* when restriction to the flow of gas is present.

Airway obstruction can occur in the anaesthetic room, during the surgical procedure in theatre, in the recovery ward and on the surgical ward post-operatively (see also Chapter 12: Extubation and Post-Operative Airway Management).

Prevention of airway obstruction is more preferable than its treatment.

- Check all equipment, including the circuit and anaesthetic machine pre-operatively.
- Use anaesthetic monitoring equipment such as spirometry, airway pressure and flow traces.
- Maintain vigilance with the surgeons encroaching on the anaesthetic equipment.

A poor capnographic trace is an indication of airway compression or complete dislodgement of the tracheal tube.

If airway obstruction should occur, initial *treatment* includes rapidly identifying and correcting the cause of the obstruction. The most common causes are:
- *Pre-induction* – abnormal anatomy (e.g. tumours, abscesses, foreign bodies).
- *Induction* – loss of pharyngeal muscle tone, abnormal positioning, laryngospasm, equipment malfunction, obstruction by a foreign body.
- *Peri-operative* – surgical misadventure, ETT kinking, ETT removal, secretions.
- *Post-extubation* – throat pack, laryngospasm, coroner's clot from behind soft palate, poor head and neck positioning, soft tissue swelling, infection, haematoma, other foreign body.

A logical sequence for the detection of the cause of the obstruction involves starting at one end of the system (e.g. common gas outlet) and working towards the other end of the system (e.g. patient's alveoli) gradually adding one piece of equipment at a time. This tests each piece of the circuit until the blocked piece has been found. If no blockage is identified in the circuit, then the blockage is either in the tracheal tube or the patient. Pass a suction catheter down the tracheal tube and consider removing it. If the tube is removed, replace it or use another airway adjunct such as a LMA to *maintain oxygenation*. If surgery is underway, maintain anaesthesia if necessary with additional intravenous agent. In this scenario, two pairs of hands are better than one so it is recommended to call for help early.

Airway soiling
Airway soiling is the process by which liquid or solid matter (e.g. blood, vomit, teeth, foreign body etc.) that is not usually present within the airway gains access to the conductive airways or alveoli. It is of

great importance to the anaesthetist as it can cause deoxygenation, airway collapse, infection etc. It is essential for the anaesthetist to be aware to what extent the operation is expected to be a dry or wet procedure. If the procedure will involve extensive irrigation or bleeding, then measures should be taken to protect the airway from soiling.

The patient's airway can become soiled pre-, peri- and post-operatively. Soiling may occur with the patient's teeth, saliva, blood, other tissue debris, surgical equipment or irrigation solutions. Local infiltration of adrenaline should reduce blood loss, as will topical vasoconstrictors such as ephedrine or cocaine. A good fitting LMA provides some protection to the trachea from debris in the oropharynx and nasopharynx. The best available method to provide protection is the inflated low-volume, high-pressure cuff of a tracheal tube in the trachea.

Consideration should be given to the insertion of a *throat pack*. This must be positioned correctly around the laryngeal inlet, not left loose in the mouth, to provide protection of the airway from soiling. A throat pack can only be used if it will not obscure surgical visualisation (therefore it is unsuitable in tonsillectomy). It is imperative that the pack be removed *prior to extubation*. Throat packs are useful even if there is an inflated cuff in the trachea, as at the level of the vocal folds there may not be an airtight seal around the tube, or accidental cuff deflation may occur. Without a pack, any liquid could seep down into the trachea before being blocked by the cuff. When suctioning the oropharynx before removing the tracheal tube, this liquid would not be removed and is then free to descend further into the airway.

In an attempt to prevent inadvertent extubation prior to the removal of a throat pack it is suggested that:
• Part of the throat pack is left hanging outside the mouth.
• A piece of sticky tape with 'throat pack' written clearly on it is stuck to the patient's forehead.
• All head and neck patients should have their vocal folds visualised by the anaesthetist while removing debris from the pharynx prior to extubation.

Bleeding tonsil
The incidence of primary haemorrhage after tonsillectomy is about 1%; the surgeon makes every effort to achieve haemostasis during the operation. However, a slipped ligature or post-operative increase in blood pressure may bring about new bleeding. In some cases, this will require a second operation. Make an assessment of airway, breathing and circulation and institute appropriate treatment (e.g. oxygen, wide-bore cannula, intravenous fluid). Replenish fluid pre-operatively if there are signs of volume depletion, but in massive haemorrhage, resuscitation is made at the same time as moving to the operating theatre.

As in any airway emergency, ensure skilled anaesthetic assistance and ask for senior help. Remember that significant amounts of blood may have been swallowed and the patient is therefore at risk of aspiration.

Two methods are proposed for airway management for induction of anaesthesia in the bleeding tonsil.

1. Inhalational induction with oxygen and vapour
This is advocated in the left lateral position and with a head down tilt. The rationale for this is that the airway is being maintained with the spontaneous respiration and blood drains away from the larynx. The problem with this method is that patient co-operation may be difficult and patient positioning for laryngoscopy and intubation is far from ideal. This is the safest method for dealing with significant ongoing bleeding.

2. Rapid sequence induction
With this method, when properly employed, there should not be any airway soiling as the cricoid pressure is applied gradually while consciousness is lost. However, because of blood in the stomach, vomiting can be triggered if the dose of induction agent was insufficient. Vomiting will necessitate release of cricoid pressure and head down tilt. The dose of the induction agent should be sufficient to allow smooth induction but not over-generous, bearing in mind the previous volume loss.

In practice, many cases of bleeding tonsils, except for brisk or torrential haemorrhage, can be managed with rapid sequence induction. If the volume status is adequate after volume resuscitation, a reasonable dose of thiopentone (4 mg/kg) can be used for rapid intravenous induction without excessive cardiovascular depression. This is followed by a standard dose of suxamethonium (1 mg/kg), and intubation undertaken with the same sized tube as that used for the previous procedure. At the end of the procedure, pass a large nasogastric tube and attempt to aspirate blood from the stomach. During recovery, protect the airway from soiling.

'Coroner's clot'
The name comes from it being discovered at post-mortem. Coroner's clot refers to a collection of blood that accumulates behind the soft palate while the patient is supine. As it is hidden from view, it may get left in post-operatively when the oropharynx is suctioned. Then, when the patient sits up or tries to inhale through their nose, it gets sucked down onto the vocal folds and can cause complete airway obstruction. After all oral and nasal procedures it is important to gently suction behind the soft palate, turning the sucker through 180°, to remove any collections that may have developed.

HEAD AND NECK, MAXILLO-FACIAL SURGERY, ENT AND NEUROSURGERY

Post–operative airway management

Extubation is covered in Chapter 12: Extubation and Post-Operative Airway Management, but there are a few points worthy of discussion in this chapter. Because of their operation, some patients will require post-operative airway protection from aspiration or airway obstruction from soft tissue swelling. These patients will require close monitoring on a ward with appropriate staff and equipment to detect and treat any post-operative airway complications. Consideration should be given to post-operative ventilation. After some major procedures, a *tracheostomy* (Figure 10.4) is performed as an alternative airway. This allows relatively easy ventilation and is well tolerated by semi-awake patients. Care of tracheostomy is a specialised area. Natural airway clearance is reduced and these patients require frequent suctioning to prevent blockage. In self-ventilating patients, oxygen administration system is attached to the 15 mm connector of the tracheostomy tube.

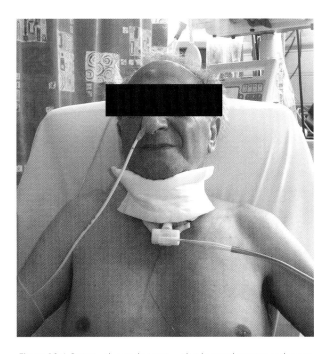

Figure 10.4 Patient with a tracheostomy with a heat and moisture exchanger.

Summary

- Team work and communication are vital to maximise safe operating conditions.
- Prevention, identification and rapid correction of airway obstruction.
- Prevention of airway soiling is a priority before, during and after the operation.
- Anticipate and prevent post-operative airway problems.

List of abbreviations

COETT	Cuffed oral endotracheal tube
ETT	Endotracheal tube
BAWO	Bilateral antral washout
EUA	Examination under anaesthetic
#	Fracture

HEAD AND NECK, MAXILLO-FACIAL SURGERY, ENT AND NEUROSURGERY

Chapter 11

The Difficult Airway

Priti Dalal

In this chapter, we will first consider what constitutes difficult airway, describe an algorithm and methods for dealing with specific difficulties, including the surgical airway and finally, deal in more detail with stridor. *The junior trainee is discouraged from attempting to anaesthetise patients where a problem is identified at assessment.*

There is no standard *definition* of the difficult airway. The report of the American Society of Anesthesiologists (ASA) Task Force on the Management of the Difficult Airway defines difficult airway as *'the clinical situation in which a conventionally trained anesthesiologist experiences difficulty with mask ventilation, difficulty with tracheal intubation, or both'.*

Mask ventilation is deemed difficult when:
- *it is not possible for the unassisted anaesthesiologist to maintain the SpO_2 >90% using 100% oxygen and positive pressure mask ventilation in a patient whose SpO_2 was >90% before anaesthetic intervention, or*
- *it is not possible for the unassisted anaesthesiologist to prevent or reverse signs of inadequate ventilation during positive pressure mask ventilation.*

Difficult tracheal intubation is said to occur if:
- *proper placement of the tracheal tube with conventional laryngoscopy requires more than three attempts, or*
- *proper insertion of the tracheal tube with conventional laryngoscopy requires more than 10 min.*

This would be mostly in cases of *difficult laryngoscopy*, when it is not possible to visualise any portion of the vocal cords with conventional laryngoscopy. This corresponds to grades III and IV of the Cormack and Lehane classification (see also Chapter 3: Routine Intubation). The trainee must bear in mind that the time spent during intubation also includes periods of oxygenation by alternative means, i.e. hand ventilation with bag, mask and airway.

The *incidence* of failed tracheal intubation is 0.05–0.33% (depending on patient population, anaesthetic skill and equipment). The higher figure refers to data from obstetric patients. The incidence of failed mask ventilation and tracheal intubation is 0.01–2.0% (similar factors as above). The reported incidence of difficult laryngoscopy is 3–13%: a difficult laryngoscopy does not always equate with difficult intubation (but also vice versa). A grade III laryngoscopic view may enable relatively easy intubation with a bougie, while a grade II with an anterior and deep lying larynx may be difficult to intubate.

Prevention and proper preparation enables the anaesthetist to deal with these situations. Adequate airway assessment (Chapter 1: Airway Assessment) is important but by no means guarantees an easy time. *Always have a primary and a secondary plan for airway management.*

THE DIFFICULT AIRWAY

The first plan must include planning for the alternative. Administer a H_2 blocker to patients at risk of aspiration, such as the morbidly obese (BMI $>35\,kg/m^2$) or those with hiatus hernia.

The ASA Task Force difficult airway algorithm (Figure 11.1) may prove useful in the management of the difficult airway.

The novice may find this algorithm slightly complicated, but with experience one may be able to understand it better. Remember not to do anything beyond your competence, hence call for help sooner rather than later. The asterisk after 'Consider calling for help' following unsuccessful 'Initial attempts at intubation' should be interpreted by the junior trainee as 'Call for help'.

Note that 'Initial attempts at intubation' include trying to optimise the laryngoscopic view, as outlined further in this chapter.

Combitube is mentioned in the algorithm described earlier as the algorithm devised by the ASA. However, this device is used little in

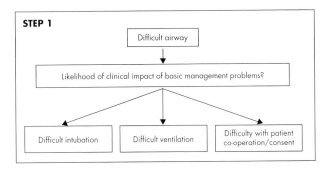

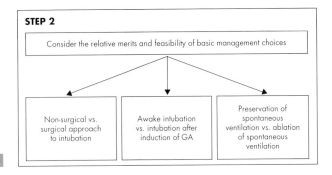

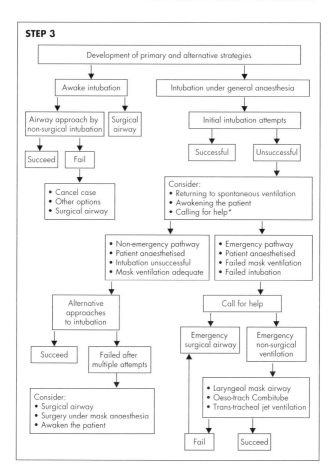

Figure 11.1 ASA Task Force difficult airway algorithm.

Britain and a practitioner not experienced with it should not attempt its use.

Difficulty with mask ventilation

A junior trainee should not administer a long acting muscle relaxant to a patient before achieving several satisfactory '*test inflations*' via the mask and airway. If ventilation is possible without muscle paralysis, it will be easier after the administration of the muscle relaxant. Try the following if there is a problem with mask ventilation at this stage:

1. Use the *correct mask fit*. Try a different size mask.

2. Try adjusting the *triple manoeuvre*: head tilt, chin lift and jaw thrust.

3. Insert the correct size oropharyngeal or a nasopharyngeal *airway*.

4. Try *two-hand* technique, i.e. the assistant squeezes the bag while the practitioner holds the mask with both hands (often needed in edentulous patients or patients of a large body mass index).

5. Use some form of *supraglottic device* such as the laryngeal mask airway (LMA).

Patients with beards may be difficult to ventilate with a mask due to a poor seal. If other difficulty is expected (e.g. the patient is obese), ask the patient to shave. Applying a gel pad with a hole for the airway may help. If unable to mask ventilate but tracheal intubation is necessary, administer suxamethonium only if no difficulty in *intubation* is expected and oxygen saturation is normal.

One must bear in mind that after induction of anaesthesia or during an inhalational anaesthetic when *airway obstruction* occurs, the patient may 'lighten' under the anaesthetic and may cough, splutter or vomit, the effect of which may be laryngospasm, bronchospasm or aspiration. It is therefore important to make an immediate diagnosis of airway obstruction and take the necessary steps to clear the airway. Make sure that the patient is adequately anaesthetised before taking control of the airway, as all the manoeuvres described above are stimulating to the patient. The anaesthetic will have to be administered intravenously, while the gas mixture is temporarily changed to 100% oxygen, plus or minus vapour, to maintain oxygenation.

Difficulty with intubation

Various anaesthetic organisations have devised their own algorithms for the management of the difficult airway. One such is the ASA algorithm as described above. *Prevention* of difficulty is preferable:

- Anticipate before the procedure – make an assessment
- Be prepared – make sure you have got all the equipment
- Spot the problem early
- Call for help early
- Do not panic – maintain oxygenation with 100% oxygen
- Have a back-up plan

Make sure the surgeon is aware of the problem.

If the patient is anaesthetised and paralysed and the *intubation is difficult* (unable to intubate with a conventional laryngoscope in the first instance) then:

1. Continue with effective mask ventilation as described above
2. Identify the problem, e.g. bucked teeth, small mouth, position of neck, large breasts (see table below)
3. Take the necessary action
4. Call for help if more than two attempts at intubation are required

Remember, the patient is safe as long as effective ventilation can be continued with 100% oxygen. If you had done test inflations you can be sure that this is possible and proceed calmly to an alternative plan. If you were not able to do a test inflation, for instance in situations of rapid sequence induction, you would have used suxamethonium and anticipate that spontaneous respiration will resume within a few minutes (the scenario of unanticipated difficult intubation and suxamethonium apnoea is fairly unlikely).

Problem	Action
Poor view (grade III–IV)	Apply or relax pressure on the larynx, alternative blade (curved/straight)
Small mouth, bucked teeth	Small blade
Large obese patient, big breasts	Short-handle or polio blade
Anterior larynx, poor view	Use a bougie/large blade, laryngeal pressure, alternative blade

Various laryngoscopic blades are available for use in different situations. The curved Macintosh blade exists in two varieties – the standard and the English type. The latter is longer, its curve is more continuous and the flange is shorter. These aspects may make laryngoscopic view better with the English type (but not necessarily the intubation). For a deep lying anterior larynx select a long and/or straight blade; for a large floppy epiglottis try the McCoy laryngoscope with a tilting tip.

At this point consider whether surgery and intubation is necessary to the conduct of the anaesthetic and surgery.

Is it an emergency or life-saving surgery?
In an emergency or life-saving surgery, one has no option other then keeping the patient anaesthetised, while maintaining spontaneous breathing or continuing effective mask ventilation until help arrives. An experienced anaesthetist may try other means of intubation if time allows, such as a fibreoptic laryngoscope, an intubating LMA, Trachlight or a Bullard laryngoscope. The latter uses a combination of fibreoptic

THE DIFFICULT AIRWAY

and mirror technology for indirect laryngoscopy without alignment. Tracheal intubation is achieved with an intubating forceps, or a stylet. If not successful and tracheal intubation is mandatory then one may have to go ahead with a surgical airway.

If it is a non-emergency surgery, the safest option is to wake the patient up and take stock. Consider the following option:

• Can the surgery be carried out under nerve blocks, central neural blockade or regional anaesthesia? If general anaesthesia is necessary then plan an alternative airway strategy or arrange for an awake fibreoptic intubation under expert guidance.

Techniques for difficult intubation
• Alternative laryngoscopes – large, McCoy or polio blade, short handle
• Intubating stylet/gum elastic bougie
• Blind nasal
• Intubating through a LMA
• Fibreoptic intubation (awake or under general anaesthesia)
• Retrograde intubation
• Surgical airway – cricothyroidotomy, tracheostomy

Difficulty with intubation and ventilation

This situation may arise during rapid sequence induction with cricoid pressure, following failure to intubate. Often the cricoid pressure applied by an inexperienced assistant contributes to the difficulty. It is very important to identify this situation early. As a part of attempts to improve the laryngoscopic view, ask the assistant to adjust or partly/fully relax cricoid pressure; watch out for regurgitation and have suction at the ready. (Further down the pathway you may need to release the cricoid pressure without the benefit of direct vision with the laryngoscope.)

If laryngoscopy and intubation have failed using strategies available, mask ventilation or LMA ventilation is the next step. Cricoid pressure should not preclude mask ventilation but other anatomical factors may make it difficult (obesity, hollow cheeks, beard). If Guedel airway/two hand ventilation does not resolve the problem, attempt laryngeal mask insertion. For this, cricoid pressure may need to be eased off or momentarily released. Ventilation should be achieved in the vast majority of patients by one of the above manoeuvres.

If all possible manoeuvres to achieve *effective ventilation* have failed, intubation is unsuccessful and the patient is desaturating, then immediate oxygen delivery to the patient is absolutely necessary. This is a *'cannot intubate, cannot ventilate'* situation. In this situation the only way to achieve oxygenation quickly, is either a trans-tracheal venti-lation using a trans-tracheal cannula, needle or surgical cricothy-roidotomy. 'Emergency tracheostomy' is not fast enough in this situation. Remember that as long as oxygenation is possible by alter-native means (mask and airway, LMA), there is no need for surgical airway.

Percutaneous needle cricothyroidotomy (Figure 11.2)
In this technique, the cricothyroid membrane is punctured vertically in the midline using a large-bore intravenous cannula (usually 14 G) attached to a syringe.

1. The patient's head is extended.
2. The cannula is advanced in the midline vertically down until air is aspirated and it is then directed caudally so that the cannula slides into the trachea and the needle is removed.
3. Aspiration of air confirms correct placement.
4. The cannula is then connected to a high pressure oxygen source (4 bar) delivering oxygen at 12–15 l/min via a Sanders jet injector (newer devices allow pressure regulation), or using some other device (Figure 11.3).

THE DIFFICULT AIRWAY

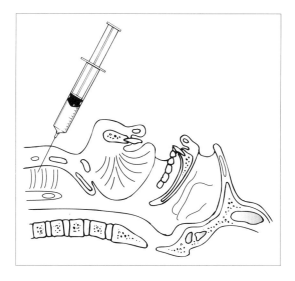

Figure 11.2 Percutaneous needle cricothyroidotomy.

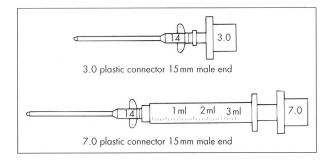

Figure 11.3 Emergency devices to connect a trans-tracheal cannula to an anaesthetic breathing system.

Advantages
1. Rapid access to the airway in acute upper airway obstruction or the 'cannot intubate, cannot ventilate situation'.
2. Buys time to prepare for a more definitive form of airway using advanced techniques.

Disadvantages
1. Trauma to surrounding structures, especially the oesophagus
2. Haemorrhage
3. Surgical emphysema
4. Pulmonary barotrauma

Surgical cricothyroidotomy (laryngotomy)
In this technique, a scalpel is used to pierce the cricothyroid membrane. It is possible to insert a small-cuffed tracheal tube or a specifically designed 4 mm cannula (Quicktrach-VBM), or a 6 mm cannula (Melker-Cook).

Trans-tracheal jet ventilation (Figure 11.4)
This technique was described in 1967. It uses the venturi principle whereby a jet of oxygen under high pressure (4 bar) entrains a larger volume of air, resulting in chest inflation. It is a potentially dangerous technique that can easily result in *barotrauma*, even with modern pressure limiting devices. It is imperative that the *upper airway is patent* to allow air entrainment and expiration; otherwise use a surgical cricothyroidotomy and a minimum 4 mm internal diameter emergency airway. This will allow ventilation with oxygen from the common gas outlet and thus limit the pressures used further.

Whatever method is used to maintain the airway, ensure that lungs are ventilated with adequate lung volumes and gas exchange is taking

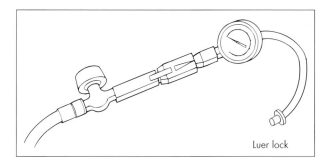

Luer lock

Figure 11.4 Trans-tracheal jet ventilation system.

place. Confirmation of tracheal tube placement is described in Chapter 3: Routine Intubation – by listening over both lung fields in the axillae and over the stomach, observing the chest rise and fall and observing the capnograph trace rise and fall with a steady plateau over several breaths.

Stridor

The ASA definition does not cover the patient with stridor. If stridor is present, it means a major upper airway obstruction/compression. Stridor is a clear warning of expected difficulty with mask ventilation and quite likely difficulty with laryngoscopy and intubation. Partial airway obstruction when the patient is conscious may rapidly progress to complete airway obstruction when consciousness is lost. The failed mask ventilation and failed intubation algorithm is of little use in this situation: the problem must be identified before anaesthesia is induced. Anticipate problems and adopt a strategy that takes into account the underlying pathology. Anaesthetising patients with major upper airway obstruction is a specialist technique – the following passage is included here for interest.

Pre-operative assessment of these patients must be thorough but expedient. If time allows, obtain CT scan to locate the obstruction and have an idea of the likely tracheal tube size that will be needed. Most patients will have had indirect laryngoscopy performed in the ENT clinic and the pathology will be identified.

Optimising breathing
Patients with major supraglottic or glottic obstruction maintain airway patency with conscious muscle effort. If a paralysing agent is administered, *complete airway obstruction* may ensue with inability to mask ventilate and very likely inability to intubate. Because air entry was already poor prior to the administration of an anaesthetic, these patients

THE DIFFICULT AIRWAY

desaturate very quickly even after long periods of pre-oxygenation. *Helium-oxygen* mixture may be useful in some of these (because of low density of helium allowing a higher turbulent flow); however, only 50% oxygen is supplied this way.

In all cases of major upper airway obstruction, the ENT surgeon must be in theatre, gowned and gloved, to provide rapid surgical access to the airway in case of failure to intubate/ventilate, by the means of a cricothyroidotomy.

Strategies for intubation
To maintain airway patency, it is vital to maintain spontaneous breathing until the point of intubation. This can be achieved in expert hands with *awake fibreoptic intubation*. However, even many senior anaesthetists will not have the degree of expertise required to negotiate a supraglottic mass with the flexible laryngoscope. Many therefore prefer *inhalational induction* of anaesthesia with oxygen and a volatile agent, maintaining spontaneous respiration until a sufficiently deep level of anaesthesia is achieved to allow laryngoscopy. Traditionally, the agent of choice was halothane, as it is relatively non-irritant and sufficiently potent. Sevoflurane has the advantage of fairly rapid induction and less sensitisation of myocardium to adrenaline. However, sevoflurane also has a rapid offset of action – a disadvantage if one has to rely solely on inhalational anaesthesia. Final choice of agent will depend on individual circumstances. MAC of at least 1.5 is necessary for laryngoscopy.

If laryngoscopy was sufficiently straightforward and saturation normal, it may be possible to use a dose of suxamethonium 1 mg/kg when anaesthesia is sufficiently deepened again after laryngoscopy. Intubation will then be accomplished after 60 s and even if mask ventilation is not possible, oxygen stores should be sufficient if saturations were normal.

In cases of severe airway obstruction, when respiration was already depressed and the anaesthetist is struggling to keep saturations above 90%, the safest option is to continue with *deep inhalational anaesthesia* until it is sufficiently deep to allow laryngoscopy and intubation without the use of muscle relaxation. If the anaesthetist is unable to maintain the airway under deep inhalational anaesthesia, the safest option is then to wake the patient up and ask the ENT surgeon to proceed with tracheostomy under local anaesthetic.

Major infraglottic (tracheal) obstruction/compression may present problems even after intubation, due to airway compression beyond the tip of the tracheal tube. The technique of choice in this situation is awake fibreoptic intubation with an uncut tracheal tube of a size determined by the narrowest point. If this technique is not available, or the tube is not long enough, emergency ventilation via Sanders injector connected to a suction catheter can provide oxygenation during sternotomy until access is obtained to both bronchi for separate ventilation of each lung. It is vital to have pressure regulation during this stage to avoid barotrauma.

The trainee anaesthetist should avoid anaesthetising patients with stridor.

Summary
- Avoid difficulty – be prepared.
- Optimise your conditions (staff, equipment, patient preparation).
- Use alternative means if primary strategy fails.
- *Oxygenate!*

Bibliography
Benumof JL. Management of the difficult airway. *Anesthesiology* 1991; 75: 531–533.

Benumof JL, Scheller MS. The importance of transtracheal JRT ventilation in the management of the difficult airway. *Anesthesiology* 1989; 71: 769–778.

Bigeleisen PB. An unusual presentation of end-tidal carbon dioxide after esophageal intubation. *Anesthesia & Analgesia* 2002; 94(6): 1534–1536.

Cossham PS. Difficult intubation. *British Journal of Anaesthesia* 1985; 57: 239.

Difficult Airway Society CD-ROM.

Dogra S, Falconer R, Latto IP. Successful difficult intubation. Tracheal tube placement over a gum-elastic bougie. *Anaesthesia* 1990; 45: 774–776.

Janssens M, Hartstein G. Management of difficult intubation. *European Journal of Anaesthesiology* 2001; 18: 3–12.

Latto JP, Vaughan RS. *Difficulties in Tracheal Intubation.* WB Saunders & Co, 1997.

Morton T, Brady S, Clancy M. Difficult airway equipment in the English emergency departments. *Anaesthesia* 2000; 55(5): 485–488.

Practice Guidelines for the Management of the Difficult Airway. A report by the American Society of Anesthesiologists Task Force on the management of the difficult airway. *Anesthesiology* 1993; 78: 597–602.

Sanehi O, Calder I. Capnography and the differentiation between tracheal and oesophageal intubation. *Anaesthesia* 1999; 54: 604–605.

Stone DJ, Gal TJ. Airway management; in Miller RD (ed.): *Anesthesia*, 5th edn. Churchill Livingstone, Chapter 39, p 1414.

THE DIFFICULT AIRWAY

Chapter 12

Extubation and Post-Operative Airway Management

Sylva Dolenska

In this chapter, aspects of recovery and how to conduct routine extubation are considered first. The post-operative airway management in some common and less common scenarios is then described and finally, common complications during recovery are discussed.

During recovery from anaesthesia, laryngeal reflexes recover, consciousness is re-gained and respiratory drive, muscle strength and co-ordination return to normal, not always in this order.

Laryngeal reflexes are obtunded in unconscious patients and this includes anaesthetised patients. They are therefore vulnerable to airway soiling from either the stomach contents, or from blood or secretions in the upper airway. Patients with residual sedation are in various stages of recovery of the laryngeal reflexes and the lower airway may not be fully protected. The reflexes of interest to the anaesthetist are the cough, gag and swallowing reflex.

Level of consciousness may be assessed using the Glasgow coma score (GCS): *GCS of 12–15 is necessary for extubation*. For patients especially at risk of airway soiling, the patient must be awake enough to respond to simple commands (opening eyes, nodding). In unconscious patients, it is possible to use monitoring. Cerebral function monitoring is available to monitor the depth of anaesthesia but is not used routinely. The monitor displays a numerical value as a percentage of complete consciousness. Eighty percent or above would indicate an 'awake' state. Another method of assessing the level of consciousness is the multiple of minimum alveolar concentration (MAC). Expired gas monitoring is now used routinely and a multiple of MAC is calculated. Note that 1.5 MAC does not equate with inspired gas concentration of 1.5%: the value displayed on the machine is a dimensionless number and represents a multiple of MAC calculated from the inspired gas mixture. For surgical anaesthesia, the level required is around 1.5 MAC. For the patient to be awake, inspired agent concentration has to decrease below 0.2 MAC (*MAC awake*).

The respiratory drive is reduced by deep inhalational anaesthesia, large doses of opioids or hypocapnia. For patients with chronic obstructive airways disease, bring the level of end-tidal CO_2 to the pre-operative level (this may be above the physiological range of 5.2–6 kPa) by reducing the minute ventilation. Adequate respiratory drive produces a respiratory rate of 10 or more.

Respiratory muscle strength may be assessed subjectively by the depth of breathing and a strong cough. The ability to sustain head lift for 5 s, or force of hand grip is also used. These tests are also partly subjective and do not test the respiratory muscles. In unconscious patients the degree of neuromuscular impairment can be assessed by using the peripheral nerve stimulator. Adequate (70% or greater) recovery of neuromuscular function occurs when on application of a train-of-four stimulus, there are four strong twitches of equal amplitude and there is no post-tetanic facilitation. For more detailed account of neuromuscular monitoring please see the reference section.

Muscle co-ordination may be impaired by a low level of consciousness or insufficient neuromuscular recovery. Signs of inco-ordination are see-sawing of the chest and abdomen, and jerky movements of face and limbs. Conscious patients may indicate double vision.

Airway management after the conclusion of surgery depends on what airway device was used, and whether the patient was breathing spontaneously or was artificially ventilated.

Routine extubation following tracheal intubation
After surgery is completed, discontinue inhalational anaesthetic and give 100% oxygen. This starts the recovery process. Giving 100% oxygen is important to prevent *diffusion hypoxia* (dilution of inspired gases in the lungs by the nitrous oxide, which leaves the bloodstream faster than nitrogen is taken up, if air is used instead of oxygen). If a non-depolarising neuromuscular blocker was used and partial or full paralysis is still present (see notes above), reverse the residual block by neostigmine 2.5 mg, given together with glycopyrrolate 0.5 mg to prevent muscarinic side-effects.

Suction the mouth and oropharynx using a wide-bore catheter such as the Yankauer sucker and suction turned to medium (20–40 cm of water). This is because during anaesthesia secretions pool in the upper airway, as laryngeal reflexes are inactive. After suction, place a Guedel airway in the mouth (if not in place already) – this prevents the patient biting the tracheal tube during recovery, thereby causing airway obstruction and inability to remove the tube later on. The airway also allows further suction of the pharynx and helps to maintain a patent airway after extubation.

A tracheal tube may be taken out only when the patient fulfils the *criteria of recovery* as discussed above, and oxygen saturation is normal.

When these criteria are all present, turn the patient on their left side (lateral to protect the airway from soiling, left so that if re-intubation is necessary, laryngoscope insertion is easy) and deflate the tracheal tube cuff gently at the end of expiration. The deflation of the cuff often produces temporary breath holding or an abnormal breathing pattern. Wait for the breathing pattern to re-establish itself before extubating, then extubate during expiration with the tracheal tube still attached to the breathing system. Just before extubation close partially the adjustable pressure limiting (APL) ('pop off') valve and squeeze the re-breathing bag to blow secretions off the larynx. Ask the assistant to apply oral suction at the same time. Immediately after extubation, apply 100% oxygen from the anaesthetic breathing system via the face-mask, with the Guedel airway still in place and observe the breathing pattern. Provided extubation was done with all criteria of recovery present, spontaneous respiration will resume – watch the movement of the re-breathing bag, as well as the chest and abdominal movement and ensure oxygen saturation is normal (95–100%). Continue to provide oxygen, or oxygen-enriched air during transfer to recovery.

Continue full *monitoring* (ECG, blood pressure, pulse oximetry) up to the point of extubation and pulse oximetry until transfer from theatre into the recovery area.

Some common scenarios
Ventilated patient at increased risk of aspiration
This scenario could include:
- Emergency surgery on a full stomach
- Patients with hiatus hernia
- Gastro-oesophageal reflux
- Morbid obesity
- ENT procedures
- Pregnancy
- Poorly controlled diabetes

See also Chapter 4: Abdominal Surgery.

At the end of the procedure, residual muscle block is reversed, inhalational anaesthetic agents discontinued and 100% oxygen given. Insert a Guedel airway if not in place. End-tidal CO_2 is brought to a usual level for the patient (this may necessitate reducing respiratory rate) and breathing is supported, usually by hand ventilation, until spontaneous respiration takes place. Spontaneous breathing may start before the consciousness returns but often the two coincide. The patient often starts coughing at this stage and the breathing pattern may be irregular. Immediately on re-awakening, the *risk of laryngospasm* is fairly high and so is the risk of airway soiling. The patient is turned into the left lateral position. Wait for the breathing pattern to become regular, with good tidal volumes and adequate respiratory rate, the return of protective reflexes (cough) and clear signs of returning consciousness (eye opening, purposeful movement – usually an attempt by the patient to remove the tube or response to command) before suctioning, deflating the tracheal tube cuff and removing the tube as described above.

Upper airway procedures
The incidence of extubation problems is high in this group (see Chapter 10: Head and Neck, Maxillo-Facial Surgery, ENT and

Neurosurgery). This may be because of the presence of blood, secretions, packs (nasal, dental, failure to remove throat pack), or high irritability of the airway in younger children. Patients with nasal packs *must* have an oral airway, as the nasal airway is blocked by the pack.

Anti-cholinergic pre-medication, particularly in young children, helps to prevent laryngospasm due to secretions. If intubated, these patients are best *extubated 'awake'*, as described above for patients at risk of aspiration. Extubating deep merely delays the onset of potential problems and the patient by that time may be in a place not well equipped to deal with them (the corridor or far corner of recovery). To blow secretions and blood off the laryngeal inlet, extubate during expiration, tightening the expiratory valve and squeezing the bag during extubation as described above. For some procedures, such as myringoplasty, it is important for the success of surgery to avoid coughing. The best method of airway management is with a laryngeal mask airway (LMA), suctioning under deep anaesthesia and removing the airway device after the return of consciousness. Judicious use of opiates and/or sedation helps to prevent undesirable emergence phenomena such as cough.

Wiring of the mandible for fractured jaw poses a particular risk to the airway after extubation. Junior trainees – senior house officers (SHOs) should not attempt to handle such cases on their own. Ensure that no pack is left behind, *wire cutters* are by the patient's head and staff know which wires may need releasing, the patient is awake and fulfils the criteria for extubation as described above. Also give a dose of an anti-cholinergic agent and a potent anti-emetic. Extubate in left lateral position, pass a soft suction catheter beyond the tip of the tracheal tube, deflate cuff and apply suction during tube removal. The nasal tube may be left in place after being partially withdrawn into the pharynx, to act as a nasopharyngeal airway. If there is a problem maintaining the airway, the wires may need to be cut. Do not wait for this until the patient is in extremis.

Ventilated patient after elective surgery – abdominal procedures
In this scenario, unless there are special risk factors mentioned above, it is reasonable to assume that the stomach is empty and the risk of airway soiling is minimal. However, muscle relaxation has to be maintained almost to the very end of surgery to enable surgical closure. Bear this in mind when administering additional boluses of muscle relaxant: ensure sufficient relaxation before closure of the peritoneum and the muscle layer but avoid if possible giving further relaxant after that. After completion of surgery, neuromuscular block may be reversed if needed. High dose neostigmine may be detrimental to bowel anastomoses due to increased tone of the smooth muscle. Therefore, use the peripheral nerve stimulator and give neostigmine, if needed, in increments. Ventilate the lungs with 100% oxygen plus the inhalational agent at concentration of about 1 MAC until spontaneous respiration

is established. The inhalational agent allows better tolerance of the tracheal tube and suctioning. Low concentration (e.g. 0.2 MAC) of the anaesthetic vapour (if used) can be used up to the point of extubation.

Ventilated patient after minor surgery outside the abdomen or thorax
There may be good reasons for paralysing and ventilating patients undergoing minor procedures, such as to prevent movement (important to ensure surgical success in microscopic surgery, or to prevent injury in instrumentation of tight spaces, e.g. retrograde pyelogram). If the patient is not at a high risk of aspiration (see above), the procedure can be done on a LMA and ventilation is continued until the surgical procedure is finished. After reversal of neuromuscular block and discontinuing the anaesthetic, recovery is usually fairly smooth if an LMA was used.

In *thyroidectomy*, whether done with a tracheal tube or an LMA, muscle relaxation and immobility are best maintained with a relatively deep general anaesthesia and generous level of MAC. At the end of the procedure, this will allow spontaneous respiration to return while the patient is still under deep inhalational anaesthesia and the vocal cords can then be inspected by direct laryngoscopy. The anaesthetist is usually asked to check the movement of both vocal cords to ensure that the recurrent laryngeal nerves are intact.

Airway devices used during recovery
Guedel (oropharyngeal) airway
A correctly chosen size will not reach the level of the larynx and therefore is relatively well tolerated. Patients will be spontaneously breathing and may remove the device when they are conscious enough to do so.

Laryngeal mask airway
The cuff of the LMA sits in the hypopharynx, with the laryngeal inlet in the middle. Correctly placed LMA will only just touch the pharyngeal side of the epiglottis, innervated by the glossopharyngeal nerve. The LMA is therefore more stimulating than the Guedel airway, but still reasonably tolerated if the patient is left undisturbed. Children, however, have a high tendency for laryngospasm and it is advocated that the LMA is removed before consciousness returns, under sufficiently deep inhalational anaesthesia. If LMA is left in place in adults, a bite block is recommended to prevent clenching of the teeth on the LMA and thus airway obstruction and/or damage to the LMA.

Patients ventilated on the LMA have a smoother recovery than intubated patients. This may be important where coughing and straining is to be avoided, e.g. following ophthalmic, ENT, plastic and neurosurgical procedures.

EXTUBATION AND POST-OPERATIVE AIRWAY MANAGEMENT

Nasopharyngeal airway

This may be used for instance during procedures using regional anaesthesia and propofol infusion for sedation. It is tolerated at a sedative,
rather than hypnotic concentration of propofol. Insertion of a nasopharyngeal airway may be traumatic due to presence of hypertrophic
turbinates or polyps; removal may then be complicated by a nose bleed.
For this reason it is best kept in place until the patient is conscious
enough to remove it by him/herself.

Tracheal tube

The presence of a tracheal tube is very stimulating as two cranial nerves
(glossopharyngeal and vagus) form the afferent arm of the laryngeal
reflexes. Laryngospasm is not an infrequent complication, particularly
after ENT surgery. Several factors co-exist at this time: inco-ordination
of laryngeal muscles (adductors overpowering the abductors), the
presence of irritants (saliva, blood, airway device) and a light plane of
anaesthesia. A tracheal tube is rarely used in recovery but in situations
where not all recovery criteria are present, for whatever reason, the
trainee anaesthetist should leave the tube in situ and stay with the
patient, supporting breathing as necessary, until the criteria for extubation are met, and seek advice from a senior colleague.

Cuff leak test

If the anaesthetist anticipates laryngeal or tracheal oedema, e.g. in
pre-eclampsia or after long tracheal intubation (>2 h), he/she should
perform a cuff leak test before extubation. When all criteria for
extubation are met, the tracheal cuff is deflated. Listen for a leak
around the tube at this point; if necessary, hand ventilate to demonstrate the leak. If no leak can be heard, laryngeal oedema is present and
difficulties can be expected: make a plan for re-intubation if breathing
should deteriorate after extubation. For the trainee, this means request-
ing senior help and *leaving the tracheal tube* in situ with anaesthesia
maintained until help is available. Further management then may
include extubating over an intra-tracheal re-intubation device, such
as the Cook airway exchange catheter (Figure 12.1), or if this is not
available, a fine bougie or a nasogastric tube is left in the trachea. These
are stimulating and sedation may be required; however, patients are
able to tolerate them when the need is explained. Extubation may
need to be delayed to allow treatment with dexamethasone, nebulised
adrenaline etc. These patients will need to be transferred to the high
dependency or critical care unit.

Complications during recovery

Airway obstruction

This will occur in the unconscious patient, if no corrective measures or
if no supraglottic airway device is used. Untreated airway obstruction

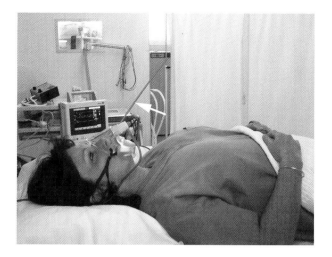

Figure 12.1 Cook airway exchange catheter in use as a re-intubation device.

leads rapidly to hypoxaemia and 3 min of hypoxaemia is sufficient to produce brain damage or death. Unconscious patients should be put in the recovery position to aid airway opening. When plastic facemasks are used, absence of water vapour on the mask in the presence of respiratory effort is a clear and early sign of airway obstruction. Cyanosis in a patient receiving oxygen therapy is a late sign. Treatment is simple, with the triple manoeuvre (head tilt, chin lift, jaw thrust), if necessary aided by the insertion of an airway. If secretions are present, they should be cleared from the mouth. Do not attempt deep suctioning as this may trigger the following complications.

Laryngospasm
This complication may happen despite the best efforts, partly because, as mentioned above, the tests of muscle strength recovery are not reliable. Laryngospasm is recognisable from a distance by crowing, or high-pitched stridor. It requires rapid correction along the lines of ABC:

- Ensure that *airway* is open (head tilt, chin lift, jaw thrust). Bilateral *jaw thrust* is particularly useful as it may physically help to open the laryngeal inlet. Suction the mouth to ensure that nothing is blocking or irritating the airway (secretions, forgotten packs). Give anti-cholinergics if secretions are a problem.
- Ensure that *breathing* and gas exchange are adequate. Administer high flow oxygen by a semi-closed anaesthetic circuit (Mapleson B,

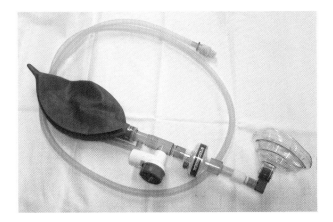

Figure 12.2 Waters' bag for use in recovery.

Waters' or re-breathing bag (Figure 12.2) if no contraindication to re-breathing, otherwise a Laerdal bag with a one way valve). Tightening the expiratory valve on the Waters' circuit will provide a degree of continuous positive airway pressure (CPAP) and help to keep the laryngeal inlet open, as well as help oxygenation. If spontaneous respiratory efforts are inadequate, try hand ventilating. This may be difficult because of the narrowed airway.

- Do not wait for deterioration in *circulation* (bradycardia from hypoxia).

If the above measures do not produce an instantaneous improvement in oxygen saturation (i.e. in less than a minute), proceed to prepare for *intubation/re-intubation*, using a small dose of intravenous induction agent and a normal dose of suxamethonium, 1 mg/kg. Give also a small dose of an anti-muscarinic agent, e.g. glycopyrrolate 0.2 mg, to prevent bradycardia due to suxamethonium and vagal stimulation by the laryngoscope. Intravenous drugs may be omitted if the patient is unconscious and cyanosed to accomplish intubation quickly (muscle tone is low at this point) but you should not wait until that stage. If oxygenation was already impaired, it is vital that the tracheal tube is passed correctly. See Chapter 3: Routine Intubation, for confirmation of tracheal tube placement.

If unsure whether intubation is possible or successful, it is better to hand ventilate with mask and airway than not ventilate at all. If the problem is still not resolved, start with fresh equipment and obtain senior help.

Bronchospasm

This complication may occur during anaesthesia in asthmatics, or as part of an anaphylactic response. High pitched wheeze over both lung fields, slow rising or no plateau on the end-tidal carbon dioxide curve and high ventilation pressures are the hallmarks. Consider alternative differential diagnosis (pneumothorax). Treatment is according to cause (bronchodilators in asthma, oxygen and adrenaline in anaphylaxis). This problem should be resolved *before* extubation, if necessary by *temporarily deepening anaesthesia* and employing the measures outlined below. Bronchospasm after extubation can be treated with nebulised salbutamol 2.5–5 mg but if severe enough to compromise oxygenation, the patient may require re-intubation plus sedation and paralysis. Salbutamol may be given intravenously in this case, at a dose of $250 \mu g$. If further bronchodilator therapy does not improve gas exchange, ventilation on the intensive therapy unit (ITU) is the next step.

Bleeding in the airway

This may happen after tonsillectomy or other intra-oral or nasal procedures (see also Chapter 10: Head and Neck, Maxillo-Facial Surgery, ENT and Neurosurgery). If the tracheal tube is still in situ, do not extubate, deepen anaesthesia and ask the surgeon to re-assess the patient. However, occasionally bleeding can occur in recovery after extubation. If brisk, place the patient in the left lateral position and slightly head down, suction the mouth, and summon the surgeon. Be careful not to suck the tonsillar bed; this would dislodge the clot which produced haemostasis. Small amounts of blood after a tonsillectomy may be due to residual blood mixed with saliva and this should resolve spontaneously. Cases of minor bleeding from the nose often respond to head elevation and an ice pack, once full consciousness has returned.

Vomiting and pulmonary aspiration

The incidence of vomiting depends on many factors. For instance it is more common in women during the second part of menstrual cycle, after certain types of surgery (gynaecological, ear or eye surgery), after recent food intake, and in patients with a history of post-operative nausea and vomiting, to name but a few of the most important causes. Emesis is an active process, which requires involuntary and voluntary muscle co-ordination. If a supraglottic airway was in place, remove it at the first sign of impending vomiting. Laryngeal reflexes are present at this stage but if the patient is not fully alert, provide additional protection of the airway by turning the patient on the side, slightly head down and suctioning. Anti-emetics may be administered intravenously as a secondary measure.

If aspiration did occur (confirm this by chest auscultation and chest X-ray), treatment is supportive: treat hypoxaemia with oxygen therapy and ensure adequate hydration. Prophylactic antibiotics should be given in cases of bowel obstruction or inhalation of other highly infective material. Severe cases may need bronchoscopy to remove the foreign material, if obstructing a major airway, and intermittent positive pressure ventilation (IPPV). Oxygen therapy and the need for transfer to ITU are determined by oxygen saturation and the clinical findings.

Hypoventilation

Hypoventilation manifests itself by signs of hypercarbia, followed by hypoxaemia. Cyanosis in a patient receiving oxygen is a late sign. Look for and treat airway obstruction and increase oxygen flow.

If breathing is still inadequate, look for signs helpful in differentiating respiratory depression (due to relative opiate overdose) from residual neuromuscular block:

- In *opiate overdose*, pupils are pinpoint even after sufficient period of inhalational anaesthetic washout (as confirmed by low MAC), respiratory rate is slow but tidal volumes are normal and train-of-four stimulation with a nerve stimulator shows strong twitches of equal height. If hypoxaemia is present, administer naloxone i.v. starting with 0.05–0.1 mg. Support the breathing by hand ventilation via Waters' bag (Figure 12.2) or Ambubag until the desired effect is produced. Too much naloxone will reverse pain relief and alternative methods of pain relief may be needed. As the duration of action of naloxone is shorter than that of most opioids used for pain relief, the patient needs to be observed for at least 20 min.

- In *residual neuromuscular block*, abnormal jerky movements of the face or upper limbs are often seen; respiratory rate may be fast and tidal volumes are small; if conscious, the patient may indicate double vision. Train of four stimulus shows a diminishing twitch size. Remember that magnesium sulphate, inhalational anaesthesia and some antibiotics all potentiate neuromuscular block. Administer a second dose of glycopyrrolate and neostigmine if hypoxaemia is present despite oxygen therapy.

Summary

1. Extubate only when all criteria of recovery are fulfilled.
2. Only self-ventilating and stable patients without a tracheal tube can be handed over to recovery staff.
3. Airway problems in recovery must be treated promptly.
4. Oxygenate! Monitor oxygen saturation continuously.
5. Call for help sooner rather than later.

Bibliography

Latto JP, Vaughan RS. *Difficulties in Tracheal Intubation*, W.B. Saunders & Co, 1997.

Index

INDEX

The text contains British terminology as in general use at the time of printing. Therefore, the terms 'adrenaline' and 'lignocaine' are used in preference to the terms 'epinephrine' and 'lidocaine'.

INDEX